Diagnosis in color

Obstetrics and Gynaecology

E. Malcolm Symonds
MD, FRCOG
**Foundation Professor of Obstetrics
and Gynaecology**
University of Nottingham

**Consultant Obstetrician and
Gynaecologist**
Queen's Medical Centre, Nottingham, UK

Marion B.A. Macpherson
DM, MRCOG
**Consultant Obstetrician and
Gynaecologist**
Queen's Medical Centre, Nottingham, UK

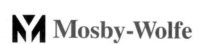

Mosby-Wolfe
London • Chicago • Philadelphia
St Louis • Sydney • Tokyo

Related titles published in Mosby's Diagnosis in color series:

The Nail in Clinical Diagnosis 2/e: Beaven & Brooks
ENT Diagnosis 3/e: Bull
Infectious Diseases 3/e: Emond, Rowland & Welsby
Surgical Diagnosis: Greig
Medical Microbiology: Hart & Shears
Breast Diseases: Mansel & Bundred
Medical Mycology: Midgley, Clayton & Hay
Skin Signs in Clinical Medicine: Savin, Hunter & Hepburn
Cardiology: Timmis & Brecker
Pediatrics: Taylor & Raffles
Oro-Facial Diseases 2/e: Tyldesley
Oral Medicine 2/e: Tyldesley
Levene's Dermatology 2/e : White:
STD & AIDS 2/e : Wisdom & Hawkins:
Physical Signs in General Medicine 2/e : Zatouroff

Publisher:	**Rebecca Whitehead**
Development Editor:	**Gina Almond**
Project Manager:	**Dave Burin**
Design:	**Greg Smith**
Cover Design:	**Lara Last**

Copyright © 1997 Times Mirror International Publishers Limited

Published in 1997 by Mosby-Wolfe, an imprint of Times Mirror International Publishers Limited

Printed in Spain by Keslan Servicios Gráficos

ISBN 0 7234 2987 1

For full details of all Times Mirror International Publishers Limited titles, please write to Times Mirror International Publishers Limited, Lynton House, 7–12 Tavistock Square, London WC1H 9LB, England.

A CIP catalogue record for this book is available from the British Library.

Contents

Acknowledgements

In this book we have attempted to collect together all the slides and photographs needed to give an overview of the common conditions observed in obstetrics and gynaecology. The majority of the photographs have been produced at the Queen's Medical Centre, Nottingham, but some images have been collected from other centres and contributors.

We are greatly indebted to the Audio-Visual Department at the Queen's Medical Centre and in particular to Mr Geoffrey Gilbert for their assistance over many years. We are also indebted to Mr Robert Hammond for providing pictures of vulval carcinomas; Mr Tony Hollingworth for his assistance with pictures in the section on cervical pathology; Dr Jane Johnson and Dr Malcolm Anderson for their assistance with pictures of gynaecological pathology; Dr Peter Twining and Mrs Jo Swallow for providing a large number of ultrasound images; Professor Brian Worthington and Mr Martin Powell for the pictures on magnetic resonance imaging; Dr Simon Fishel for providing the embryology pictures and Dr Norman Thomas who both performed and photographed the anatomical prosections. Dr Derek Johnson provided pictures of some of the congenital anomalies. We are also indebted to Mr Marcus Filshie and Mr Martin Powell for the pictures of minimal invasive surgery.

Finally, we owe a great debt of gratitude to all those patients who so kindly agreed, albeit anonymously, to appear in print. Although care has been taken to ensure anonymity, the authors apologise for any oversight in this regard.

We hope that readers get some information from the wide range of pictures and pathologies. Although the book contains over 400 pictures, it is by no means comprehensive. Like all such works, it bears the hallmark of the authors' preferences, but we hope it will provide a firm pictorial basis for obstetrics and gynaecology in both undergraduate and postgraduate studies.

Marion B.A. Macpherson, DM, MRCOG
E. Malcolm Symonds, MD, FRCOG

Preface

Obstetrics and gynaecology are generally visual subjects. They lend themselves well to illustrative material. Indeed, gynaecological pathology often has a spectacular dimension and the appearances of any tumour lend themselves well to the visual memory.

We compiled this book as a combined photographic record, bearing in mind that many students have limited time in which to study this subject in medical school. It is also presented as an aid to practising clinicians to remind them of common conditions of pregnancy and of gynaecological pathology. The collection is by no means comprehensive. It must be taken as complementary to other presentations which limit the subject to one specialised topic.

Some of the photographs have been collected over the last 20 years, but the majority of the obstetric presentations are more recent.

Nothing can suitably illustrate obstetric procedures in a static form, but these images, if considered in conjunction with line drawings, provide a useful reminder and illustration of common obstetric procedures.

The ovaries, because of their totipotential nature, produce a wide variety of benign and malignant tumours. No attempt has been made to amass a comprehensive collection. Furthermore, many tumours have an appearance that can only be diagnosed histologically and it has not been our intention to present this book as a histology text.

Some surgical techniques have been included to illustrate the pathology or structural abnormalities of the genital tract better and provide photographic material of common procedures that can be used to educate both practitioners and patients.

Marion B.A. Macpherson, DM, MRCOG
E. Malcolm Symonds, MD, FRCOG

1 Methods of examination

Obstetrics

Pregnancy produces changes in every system in the body in the process of achieving preparation for parturition and the support of the newborn child. Some of these changes are obvious and readily apparent and others are of a more subtle nature and are less specific.

At the initial visit to clinic, a complete physical examination is performed. Height is recorded and the weight is recorded at the first and all subsequent visits. Blood pressure is recorded with the patient supine and in the lateral supine position to avoid vena caval compression (**1.1**). Diastolic blood pressure

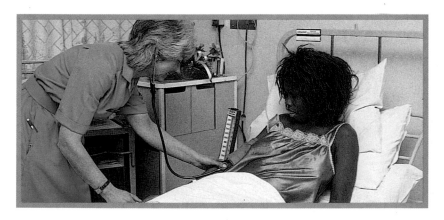

↑ 1.1 Blood pressure is recorded from the right arm

Cuff size is important. Posture should be consistent and blood pressure is usually taken with the mother lying supine with a left lateral tilt to relieve any pressure of the enlarged pregnant uterus from the inferior vena cava. The diastolic blood pressure in pregnancy is recorded as the fourth Korotkoff sound.

is usually taken as the Korotkoff fourth sound, although there has been some recent shift to recording values that relate to the disappearance of the sound.

Skin pigmentation (**1.2**) is most noticeable on the forehead and the cheeks, particularly in women of darker complexion and from sunny climates.

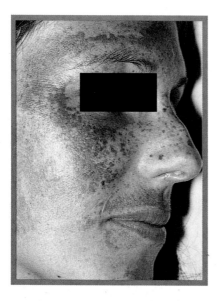

← 1.2 Chloasma—the 'mask of pregnancy'

Pigmentation occurs across the forehead and the cheeks in some women during pregnancy and later disappears.

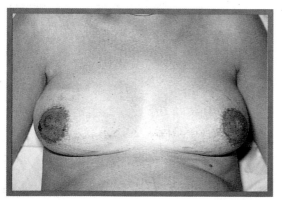

← 1.3 Breast changes in pregnancy

These include enlargement, increased vascularity, and the production of colostrum.

Breast changes include an increase in size and vascularity as well as increased areolar pigmentation and the development of Montgomery's tubercles (**1.3–1.5**).

→ 1.4 The areola of the nipple

This shows increased pigmentation and the development of raised sebaceous glands known as Montgomery's tubercles.

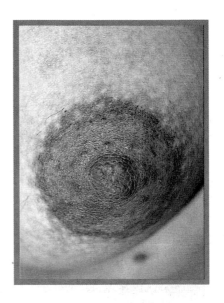

→ 1.5 The areola

This shows marked pigmentation in women with dark skins.

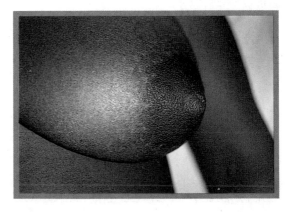

Striae gravidarum do not become apparent on the abdomen, thighs and breasts of all pregnant women, but may be particularly florid in some women, leaving silvery abdominal scars after the pregnancy (**1.6–1.7**).

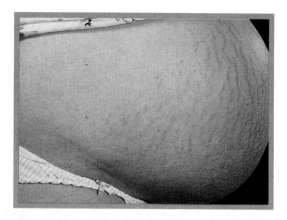

← 1.6 Lateral inspection of the abdomen in advanced pregnancy

This shows the presence of striae gravidarum, which extend onto the breasts and the lateral surface of the thighs and buttocks.

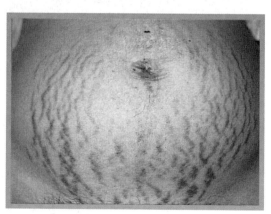

← 1.7 Direct view of the anterior abdominal wall in the third trimester of pregnancy

The scars are initially purplish in colour and appear in lines of stress in the skin. In subsequent pregnancies, the scars are silvery white in appearance.

Abdominal examination is particularly important in assessing fetal growth and development. Serial measurements of fundal height allow a reasonable measurement of fetal growth (**1.8–1.10**).

→ 1.8 Palpation of the uterine fundus at 18 weeks' gestation

The border of the hand is placed along the superior margin of the uterine fundus.

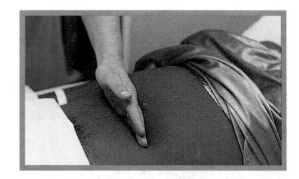

→ 1.9 By 36 weeks' gestation

The uterine fundus lies in apposition to the xiphisternum.

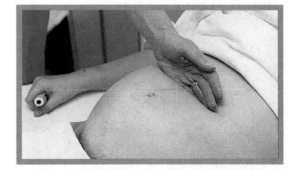

→ 1.10 Measurement of the fundal height allows assessment of gestational age and fetal size

Serial measurements are particularly useful in the assessment of fetal growth.

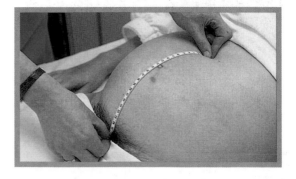

Palpation of the fetal parts enables determination of fetal lie, presentation and attitude, as well as the station of the presenting part (**1.11–1.14**).

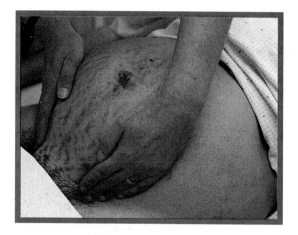

← 1.11 Palpation of the presenting part and the position of the back

These are important routine observations.

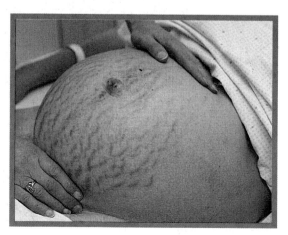

← 1.12 Pawlik's grip

This enables the attendant to assess the degree of descent of the presenting part. It should be used with gentleness because, if applied roughly, it may be uncomfortable for the mother.

→ 1.13 Checking for the presence of excessive amniotic fluid or hydramnios

This involves eliciting the presence of a fluid thrill. A hand placed centrally dampens down vibrations in the subcutaneous fat.

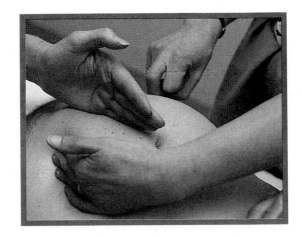

→ 1.14 Auscultation of the fetal heart

The Pinard stethoscope is applied firmly at right angles to the abdominal wall. The instrument should not be held in the hand during auscultation because this may muffle the sound.

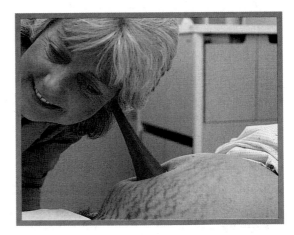

Pelvic examination

At the first visit, a pelvic examination is performed to exclude any pathology and to assess the size and position of the uterus. Pregnancy induces marked changes in the vaginal walls with increased vascularity and transudation (**1.15**). The cervix also undergoes enlargement, softening and increased vascularity.

Assessment of the bony pelvis involves palpation for the sacral promontory (**1.16**), observation of the sacral curve (**1.17**), and identification of the ischial spines (**1.18**), the angle of the subpubic arch (**1.19**), and the intertuberous diameter. Urine analysis is performed at each antenatal visit and tested for protein, glucose and ketone bodies.

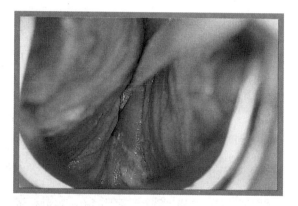

← 1.15 Speculum examination

This reveals the increased vascularity and engorgement of the vaginal walls in pregnancy.

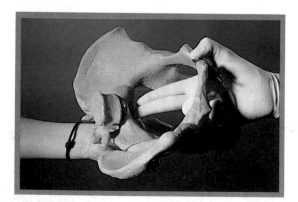

← 1.16 Assessment of the bony pelvis

Feeling for the sacral promontory allows an assessment of the anteroposterior diameter of the pelvic inlet.

→ 1.17 Palpation of the sacral curve and the attitude of the coccyx

This is important in the assessment of the pelvic cavity.

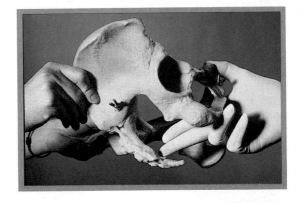

→ 1.18 The ischial spines represent the lateral limits of the narrowest plane in the pelvis

The top of the finger can be seen in apposition to the right ischial spine.

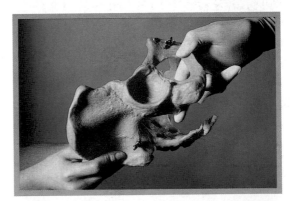

→ 1.19 The normal subpubic angle is 90°

A narrow subpubic angle indicates both a narrow pelvic outlet and often a funnel pelvis.

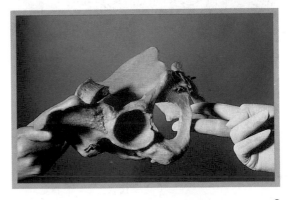

The gynaecological examination

The approach to any clinical problem in any discipline in medicine involves obtaining a detailed medical and surgical history as well as a detailed history of the presenting complaint. Examination of a patient presenting with gynaecological symptoms also involves a general examination with particular assessment of the breasts (**1.20–1.23**) and abdomen (**1.24**).

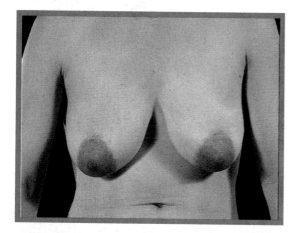

← 1.20 Inspection of the breasts

This should be a routine part of the gynaecological examination.

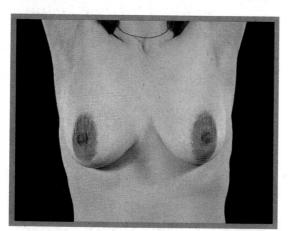

← 1.21 The breast should be systematically inspected

The position and mobility of any breast lumps can then be defined.

→ 1.22 Palpation of the inner quadrants of the breast

This should form part of a systematic routine.

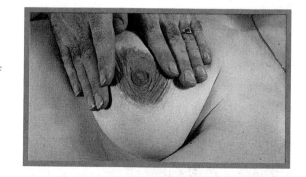

→ 1.23 Palpation of the axillary tail

This is particularly important as assessment must include all breast tissue.

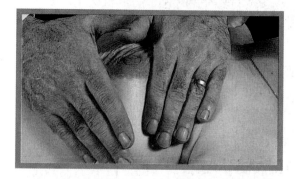

→ 1.24 Examination of the abdomen may show distension

A view from a lateral aspect, as in this case, shows the outline of a large ovarian cyst with central dullness to percussion.

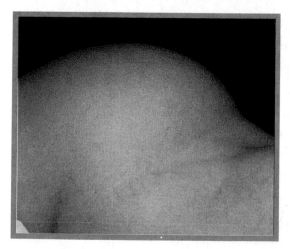

Pelvic examination

Pelvic examination (**1.25–1.31**) involves speculum inspection and bimanual examination. Both procedures are equally important.

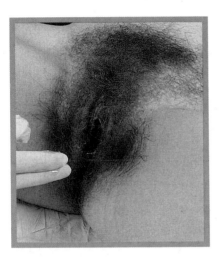

← 1.25 Inspection of the vulva

Pelvic examination involves inspection of the vulva. Look for vulval lesions and note the general condition of the vulval skin.

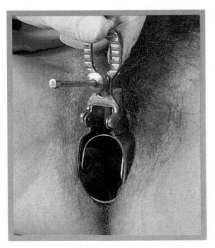

← 1.26 Inspection of the vaginal walls

Insertion of a bivalve or Cuscoe's speculum allows inspection of the vaginal walls.

- A cervical smear is taken where appropriate after inspecting the cervix (see **1.27–1.29**).
- Bimanual examination (see **1.30**) is used to assess the size, shape, and position of the uterus, and the presence of any adnexal tumours.

The essence of good pelvic examination is to obtain the maximum information with minimal discomfort.

→ 1.27 Inspection of the cervix

Insertion of a bivalve or Cuscoe's speculum also allows inspection of the cervix.

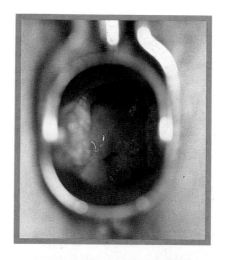

→ 1.28 Cervical smear

A cervical smear is taken with an Ayre's speculum.

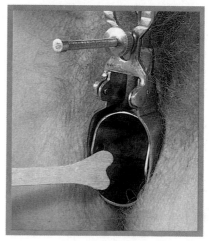

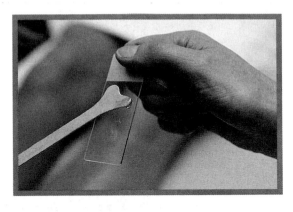

← 1.29 Cervical smear

The material obtained by scraping the cervix is placed on a glass slide for fixation and staining.

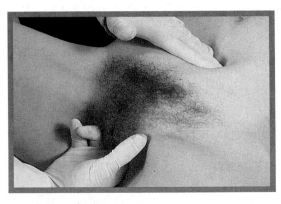

← 1.30 Bimanual palpation of the pelvic organs

The pelvic examination is completed by bimanual palpation of the pelvic organs. Palpation of the fornices is important to detect adrenal masses.

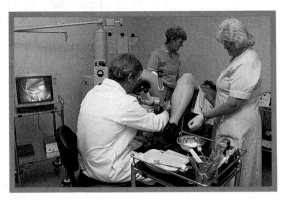

← 1.31 Colposcopy

Sometimes a more detailed examination of the cervix is indicated. A colposcope allows a close inspection of cervical epithelium.

2 Fetoplacental growth and development

Fertilisation occurs when spermatozoa reach the oocyte (**2.1–2.6**) in the ampulla of the tube. After the nucleus of the sperm head passes into the cytoplasm of the oocyte, the second polar body of the oocyte is expelled.

As the conceptus passes down the tube, it undergoes cleavage (**2.7–2.9**) and, at the 16-cell stage, forms the morula and then the blastocyst (**2.10–2.12**). Implantation occurs six days after ovulation. Subsequent development of the fetus occurs initially as the result of a massive increase in the number of cells in the inner cell mass, but with relatively little increase in the mass.

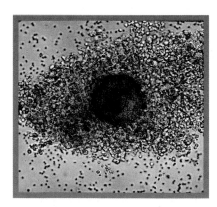

↑ **2.1 The oocyte/cumulus complex**

At the moment of aspiration from a human Graafian follicle.

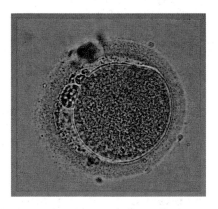

↑ **2.2 An unfertilised egg in metaphase II**

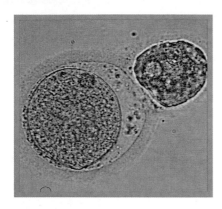

← 2.3 A bi-ovular zona pellucida or a fused zona pellucida containing two oocytes

One oocyte appears to be mature, but the other contains a germinal vesicle and is slightly degenerate.

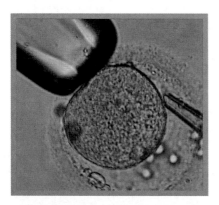

← 2.4 Subzonal insemination

The injection of spermatozoa into the perivitelline space is facilitated by slightly dehydrating the oocyte. Microinjection is performed with a needle 11 microns in diameter and a holding pipette about 30 microns in diameter.

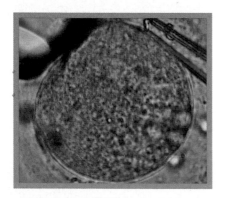

← 2.5 Micro-injection

High magnification view.

→ 2.6 A one-cell egg with sperm in the perivitelline space

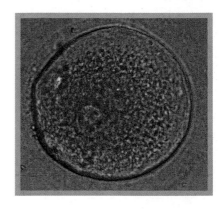

→ 2.7 A two-cell pronucleate human oocyte

18 hours after insemination *in vitro*.

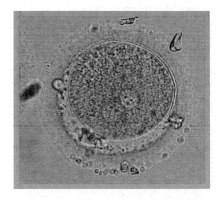

→ 2.8 A three-cell pronucleate human oocyte with several attendants on the surface of the zona pellucida

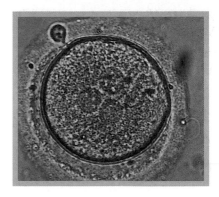

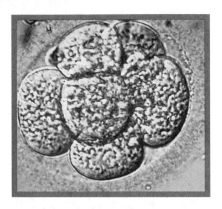

← 2.9 A six-cell human embryo

49 hours after insemination *in vitro.*

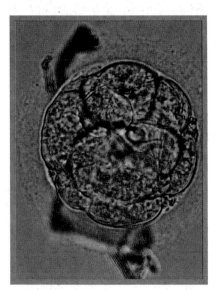

← 2.10 Early human morula

74 hours post insemination *in vitro.*

→ 2.11 A late human morula and blastocyst

Note the small cavitation and presence of blastocoelic fluid in the late morula and the full blastocoelic cavity and inner cell mass.

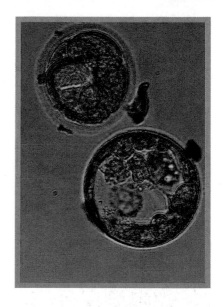

→ 2.12 Blastocyst

High-power view at 5.5 days post insemination.

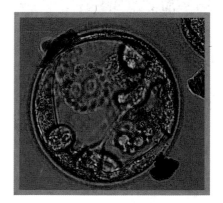

The major processes of organogenesis are complete by 12 weeks' gestation (**2.13**), but the development of function in the various systems continues at different rates. There is a heartbeat by five weeks' gestation and fetal respiration is established *in utero* by 12 weeks. Mucosal glands appear in the gut by 16 weeks (**2.14–2.15**) and by 26 weeks most of the digestive enzymes are present. Functional development of the fetal kidney favours early development of the renal tubules before glomerular function occurs and fetal urine makes a significant contribution to amniotic fluid.

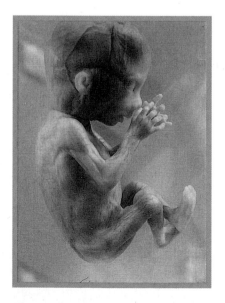

← 2.13 At 12 weeks' gestation

The fetus reacts to stimuli. The upper limbs reach their final relative length and the fetal sex is distinguishable externally.

→ 2.14 At 16 weeks' gestation

Crown–rump length is 122 mm. Lower limbs achieve their final relative length and the eyes face anteriorly.

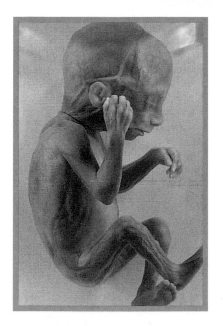

→ 2.15 At 24 weeks' gestation

The fetal lungs have started to secrete surfactant.

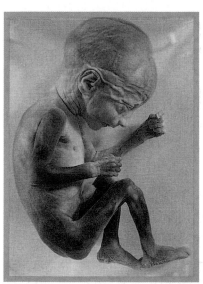

Placenta

The placenta has a vital function in gaseous exchange, fetal nutrition, and the manipulation of maternal physiology to the advantage of the fetus. The functional unit of the placenta is the stem villus. These develop from the chorion frondosum and the remaining 'non-placental' portion of the chorion frondosum eventually forms the chorion laeve as part of the fetal membranes (**2.16**). The amnion lies inside the chorion and is loosely attached to it (**2.17**).

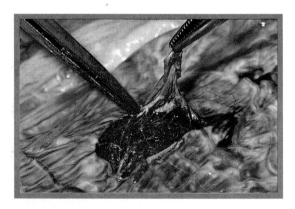

← 2.16 The fetal surface of the placenta

This shows the chorionic plate and the fetal vessels.

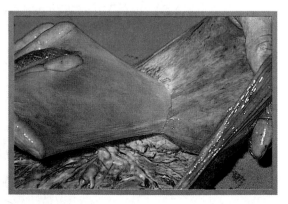

← 2.17 The fetal membranes

These consist of the two layers of chorion and the amnion.

The maternal surface of the placenta exhibits a series of cotyledons (**2.18–2.21**), which are clusters of fetal villi. At term the mature placenta weighs approximately 600 g. The cotyledon may become infarcted (**2.22**) and if this occurs in sufficient numbers fetal growth is impaired. The umbilical cord contains two arteries and one vein surrounded by Wharton's jelly and amnion. The vessels have a helical disposition.

→ 2.18 Maternal surface of the full-term placenta

This shows the cotyledonary structure.

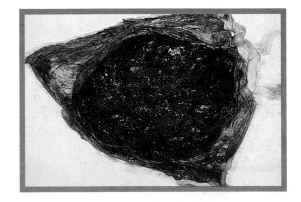

→ 2.19 Fetal surface of a circumvallate placenta

There is reduplication of the membrane at the rim of the placenta.

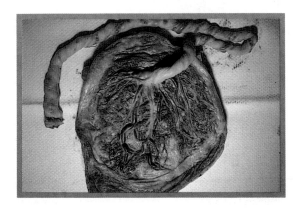

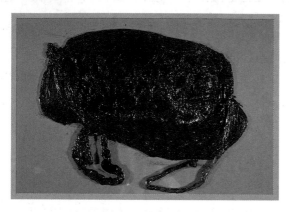

← 2.20 Placental abruption

This leaves the maternal surface covered with blood clot.

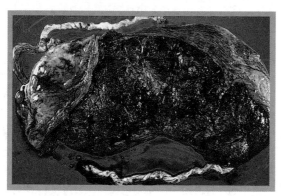

← 2.21 A twin placenta

A twin placenta with fusion of the two placentae, which appear to be indistinguishable. The two umbilical cords can be seen.

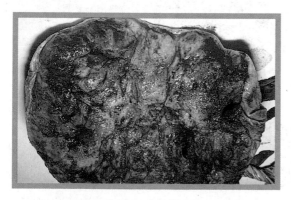

← 2.22 Placenta showing multiple white infarcted cotyledons

These affect nearly half the placental surface.

3 | Congenital abnormalities and prenatal diagnosis

The incidence of major congenital abnormalities varies from country to country. In the UK, the figure has been estimated at 25–30/1000 births.

Prenatal screening

Prenatal screening (**3.1–3.9**) includes:
- Biochemical tests such as alpha fetoprotein, combined alpha fetoprotein, HCG and serum oestriol.
- Chorion villus sampling.
- Amniocentesis
- Ultrasound screening, now the major technique for imaging structural abnormalities.

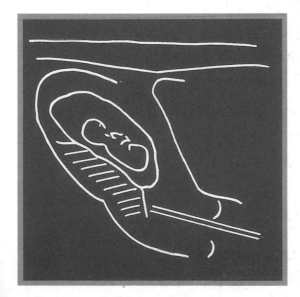

← 3.1 Chorion villus sampling

Schematic representation of chorion villus biopsy. A small sample of chorionic tissue is taken either vaginally through the cervix or via the abdominal route.

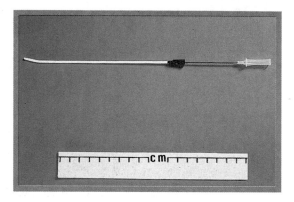

←3.2 Chorion villus sampling

Chorion villus sampling needle.

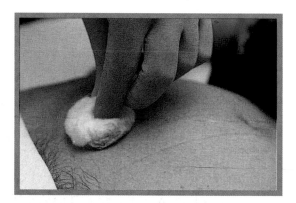

←3.3 Amniocentesis

Preparation of the maternal anterior abdominal wall for amniocentesis.

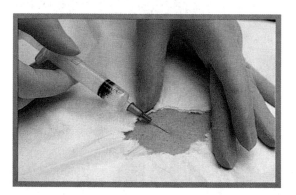

←3.4 Amniocentesis

Infiltration of local anaesthetic over the placement site of the amniocentesis needle.

→ 3.5 Amniocentesis

Insertion of the amniocentesis needle into a pool of amniotic fluid detected by ultrasound.

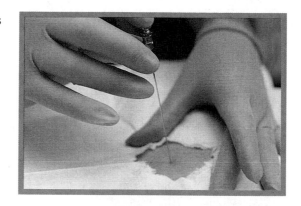

→ 3.6 Amniocentesis

Aspiration of amniotic fluid with a 20 ml syringe.

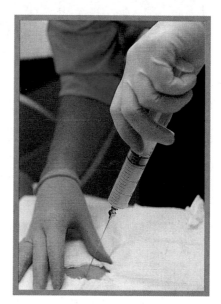

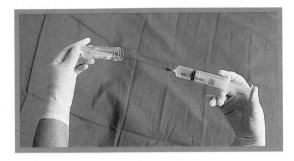

← 3.7 Amniocentesis

Alliquoting of the amniotic fluid for cell culture and biochemistry.

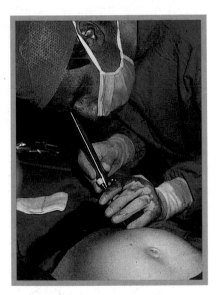

← 3.8 Fetoscopy

Direct visualisation of the fetus through an endoscope is now rarely used.

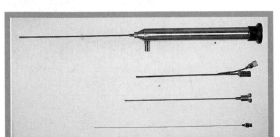

← 3.9 Fetoscopy

Needle endoscope used for fetoscopy.

Most common congenital abnormalities

The five most common groups of congenital abnormalities (**3.10–3.24**) include:
- Neural tube defects.
- Congenital heart disease.
- Severe mental retardation.
- Down's syndrome.
- Hare lip/cleft palate.

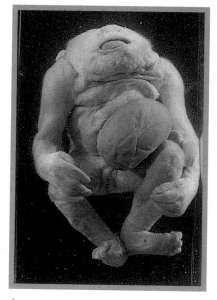

↑ **3.10 Anencephaly**

The cerebral hemisphere and cranial vault are absent.

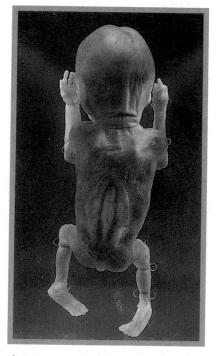

↑ **3.11 Lumbar myelomeningo-coele**

The defect in the posterior bony aspect of the vertebrae exposes the spinal membranes.

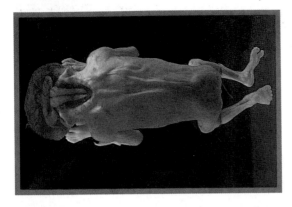

← 3.12 Meningo-myelocoele of the cervical spine

A similar defect high in the spinal canal.

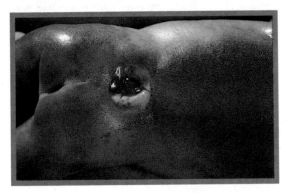

← 3.13 Small open neural tube defect

This was identified by high amniotic fluid alpha fetoprotein levels and confirmed at the time of abortion.

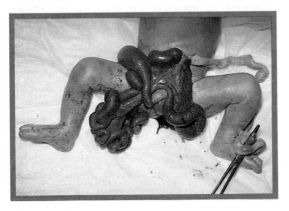

← 3.14 Gross exom-phalus

Shortly after delivery of a mature infant by Caesarean section.

→ 3.15 Gross exomphalus: successful closure of the abdominal wall defect

This was performed immediately after delivery.

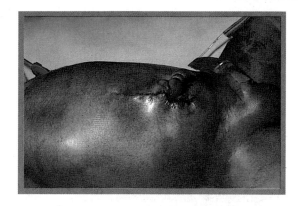

→ 3.16 Large encephalocoele

Lateral view.

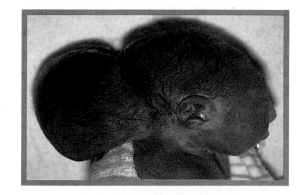

→ 3.17 Large encephalocoele

Posterior view.

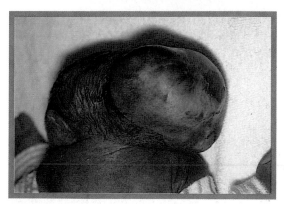

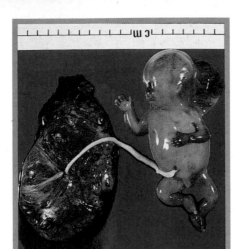

↑ **3.18 Large cystic hygroma**

This was detected by ultrasound scan.

↑ **3.19 Grossly hydropic fetus associated with trisomy**

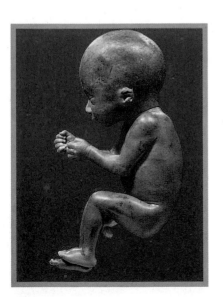

← **3.20 Potter's syndrome**

This syndrome is associated with renal agenesis and is incompatible with life when there is complete renal agenesis. The 'crumpled ears' reflect poor cartilage development and the effects of severe oligohydramnios.

→ 3.21 Down's syndrome

Facial appearance of an infant with Down's syndrome. (Courtesy of Dr. D.I. Johnston.)

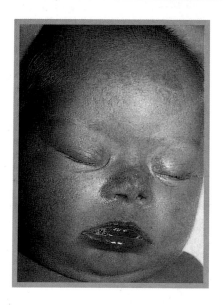

→ 3.22 Turner's syndrome

This syndrome is associated with pedal and lower limb oedema and chromosome analysis of 45XO.

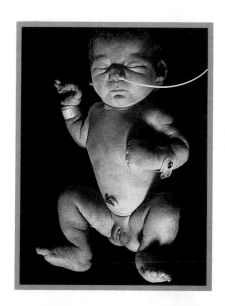

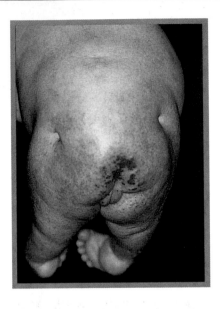

← 3.23 Caudal regimen syndrome (sacral agenesis) in an infant of a diabetic mother

(Courtesy of Dr. D.I. Johnston.)

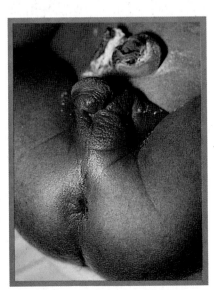

← 3.24 Congenital adrenal hyperplasia (21-hydroxylase deficiency)

This female infant shows clitoromegaly and labio- scrotal fusion. (Courtesy of Dr. D.I. Johnston.)

4 | Medical disorders
of pregnancy

The majority of medical complications encountered in pregnancy do not present with physical signs. However, some common conditions are shown in this brief section (**4.1–4.10**). Most of the medical conditions do not exhibit any specific visual signs and cannot therefore be represented macroscopically by visual images.

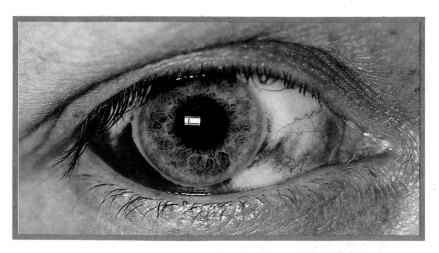

↑ 4.1 Subconjunctival ecchymosis following normal delivery

The rupture of subconjunctival vessels follows the straining that occurs in the second stage of labour.

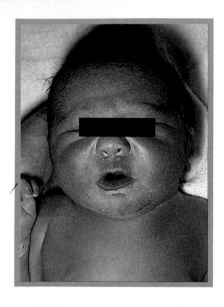

← 4.2 Macroscopic features of an infant born to a mother with insulin-dependent diabetes

The child has increased subcutaneous fat and generalised visceromegaly.

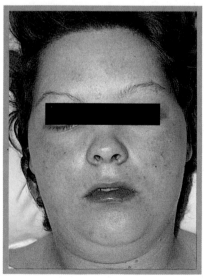

← 4.3 Facial oedema and severe pre-eclampsia

Oedema commonly occurs in the limb extremities, over the face, and the abdominal wall.

→ 4.4 Facial oedema and severe pre-eclampsia

Lateral view.

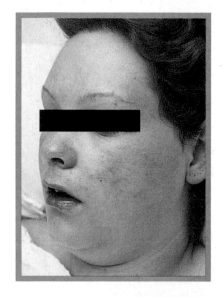

→ 4.5 Thyroid enlargement in a normal pregnancy

Some degree of goitre is physiologically normal.

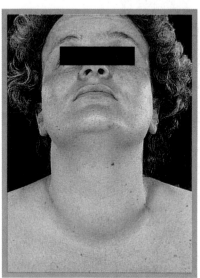

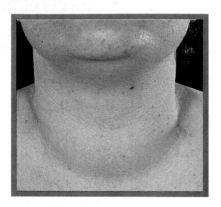

← 4.6 Thyroid enlargement

Close up view.

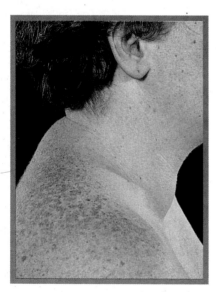

← 4.7 Thyroid enlargement

In profile. It is often difficult to differentiate between normal and abnormal thyroid enlargement in pregnancy.

→ 4.8 Herpes gestationis on the abdomen

This is a rare condition that arises only during pregnancy and disappears after delivery.

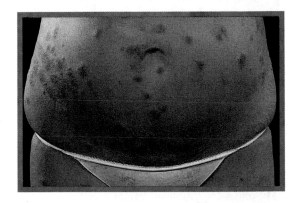

→ 4.9 Herpes gestationis on the abdomen

Lateral view.

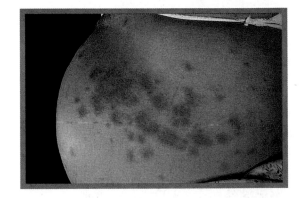

→ 4.10 Herpes gestationis on the thigh

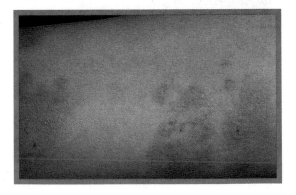

5 | Antepartum and intrapartum monitoring

Antepartum and intrapartum monitoring are standard techniques of fetal assessment.
- Antenatally, the fetal heart rate is monitored by pulsed Doppler ultrasound (**5.1–5.5**).
- During the course of labour, fetal heart rate can be monitored directly by applying an electrode to the fetal presenting part using the fetal ECG. The heart rate and uterine activity are recorded and the heart rate is displayed in an analogue tracing so that patterns of heart rate change can be identified (**5.6–5.13**). More recently, techniques have been developed to show the features of the fetal ECG waveform in real time displays.

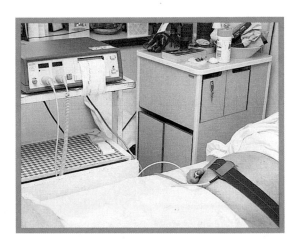

← 5.1 Standard antenatal cardio-tocography (CTG)

The transducers are applied to the maternal abdomen to detect the fetal heart beat and uterine contractions.

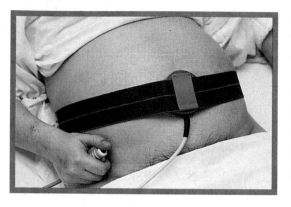

← 5.2 Standard antenatal CTG

The application of the heart rate transducer attached to the maternal abdominal wall. The mother clasps the event marker in her right hand and presses the button when she feels a fetal movement.

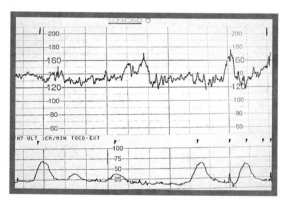

← 5.3 Normal antenatal CTG

This shows baseline variability of greater than 5 beats/minute.

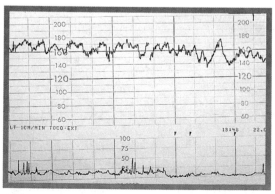

← 5.4 Antenatal CTG showing a resting tachycardia with normal baseline variability

→ 5.5 Antenatal CTG with a normal baseline heart rate, but no baseline variability

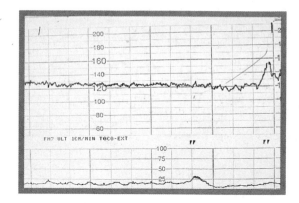

→ 5.6 Copeland electrode

The Copeland electrode is used for direct application to the fetal presenting part in labour.

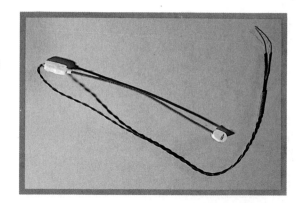

→ 5.7 Copeland electrode

Single coil of the Copeland disposable electrode.

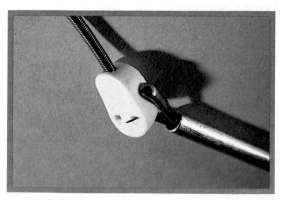

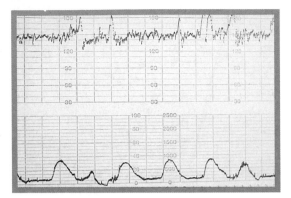

← 5.8 Normal intrapartum recording

This shows a normal baseline heart rate and normal baseline variability. The uterine contractions can be seen on the bottom line.

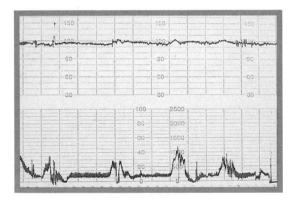

← 5.9 Baseline bradycardia with loss of heart rate variability during the first stage of labour

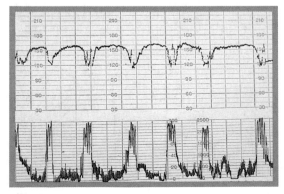

← 5.10 Early decelerations

The peak of the deceleration coinciding with the zenith of the uterine contraction.

→ 5.11 Profound and persistent bradycardia with slow recovery to a normal heart rate

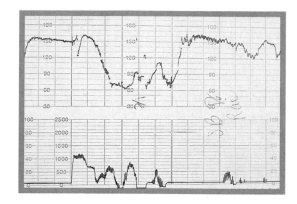

→ 5.12 Variable decelerations

These do not appear to be related to the uterine contractions.

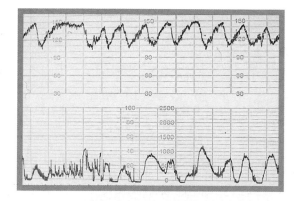

→ 5.13 Complications of a fetal scalp electrode

This shows two ulcerated areas associated with hair loss.

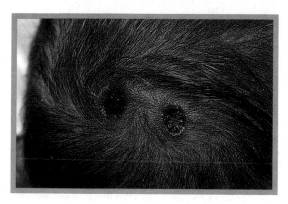

These techniques have been developed in an attempt to detect fetal asphyxia. Fetal acid–base balance can be measured directly in labour by sampling scalp blood taken from the presenting parts (**5.14–5.16**).

The baseline heart rate is the number of beats per minute between alterations, and lies between 120 to 160 beats/minute. Fetal heart rate (FHR) variability is defined as the amplitude of oscillations of the baseline, and where it is greater than 5 beats/ minute, it is considered to be normal. An amplitude of between 3–5 beats/minute is often associated with sleep patterns, and is only significant if associated with other FHR abnormalities. A flat baseline with a variability of 0–2

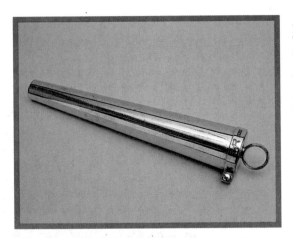

← 5.14 Sampling fetal scalp blood: the amnioscope

This is introduced through the cervical os to display the fetal presenting part. It consists of an obturator and a cannula.

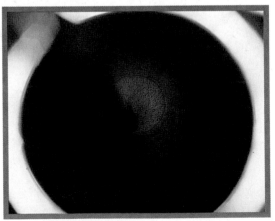

← 5.15 Sampling fetal scalp blood

A sharp blade is introduced on a long holder to incise the scalp.

beats/minute, when associated with other abnormalities, is considered ominous.

Alterations in the FHR lasting less than 10 minutes include accelerations which are indications of good fetal prognosis and decelerations which may be early, late or variable. The definition is based on the time relationship to uterine contractions. The lag time is defined as the interval between the peak of the contractions and the nadir of the decelerations. In an early deceleration, the lag time is less than 18 seconds; in the late deceleration it is greater than 18 seconds. Some examples of antenatal CTGs are demonstrated (**5.3–5.5**), and Figures **5.8–5.12** show examples of intrapartum recordings.

→ 5.16 Sampling fetal scalp blood

A drop of blood can be seen to form on the fetal scalp and can then be aspirated into a fetal capillary and submitted for fetal acid–base balance measurement.

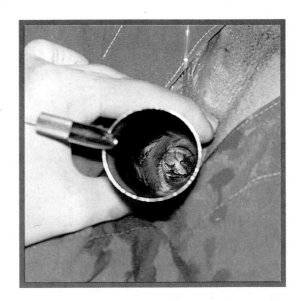

6 Spontaneous vaginal delivery and breech delivery

Spontaneous vaginal delivery

Normal spontaneous vaginal delivery (**6.1–6.9**) is associated with progressive flexion and descent of the head, distension of the pelvic floor, delivery of the head, restitution and external rotation and delivery of the shoulders and trunk. Placental delivery is achieved by cord traction and fundal pressure.

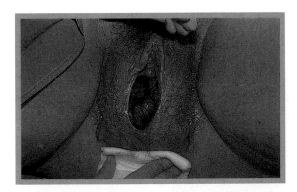

← 6.1 Spontaneous vaginal delivery: the second stage of labour

The scalp becomes visible with contractions and expulsive efforts by the mother.

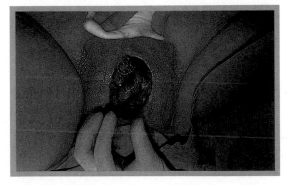

← 6.2 Spontaneous vaginal delivery: crowning of the head

The perineum is distended until the head crowns.

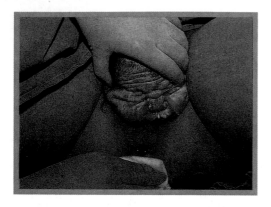

← 6.3 Spontaneous vaginal delivery: at delivery

The head is in the anteroposterior position at delivery.

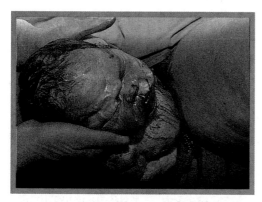

← 6.4 Spontaneous vaginal delivery: delivery of the head and shoulders

Delivery of the head is accompanied by external rotation so that the occiput rotates from the anterior position to a point laterally. The anterior shoulder is delivered by downward traction on the head and the posterior shoulder by anterior traction.

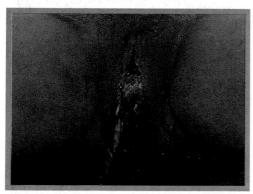

← 6.5 Spontaneous vaginal delivery: the third stage of labour

The abdomen is palpated to make sure that the uterine fundus is contracted. The placenta appears distending the vulva.

→ 6.6 Spontaneous vaginal delivery: placental delivery

The placenta is delivered with cord traction and counter pressure against the uterine fundus.

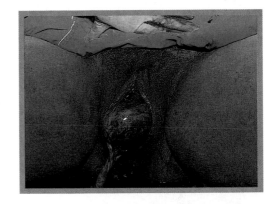

→ 6.7 Spontaneous vaginal delivery: after delivery

The cord is clamped and cut and the infant is weighed.

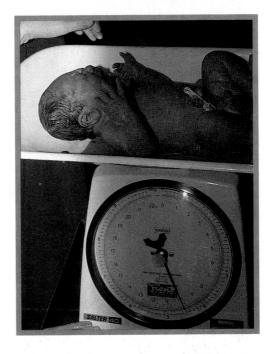

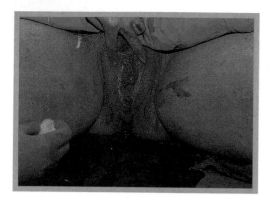

← 6.8 Spontaneous vaginal delivery: after delivery

The perineum, vulva, and vaginal wall are checked for lacerations.

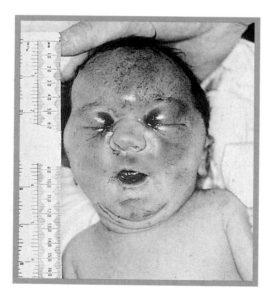

← 6.9 Spontaneous vaginal delivery: face presentation

Abnormal facial bruising followed spontaneous vaginal delivery as a face presentation.

Breech delivery

In a breech presentation (**6.10–6.26**), the buttocks are expelled to the waist, the limbs are lifted out by flexion of the thighs and knees and the trunk is allowed to hang until the head enters the pelvis.

Delivery of the head is achieved by anterior rotation of the trunk and the application of forceps to the aftercoming head.

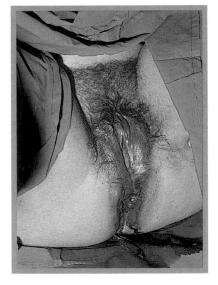

↑ 6.10 Breech delivery: breech presentation

The anterior buttock appears at the introitus.

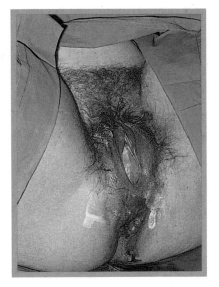

↑ 6.11 Breech delivery: breech presentation

The vulva and anus are distended by the breech.

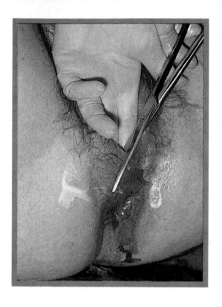

← 6.12 Breech delivery: episiotomy

A mediolateral episiotomy is cut to facilitate descent of the breech and subsequent delivery of the fetal head.

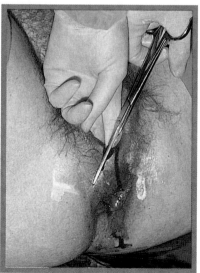

← 6.13 Breech delivery: episiotomy

Care is taken not to injure the presenting part.

→ 6.14 Breech delivery: fetal descent

Further descent of the anterior buttock occurs.

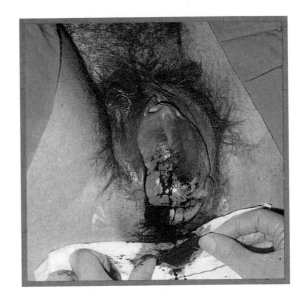

→ 6.15 Breech delivery: fetal descent

Both buttocks come into view as well as the anterior thigh.

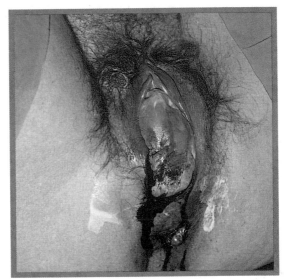

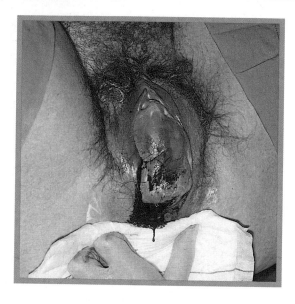

← 6.16 Breech delivery: fetal descent

The fetal anus and vulva are now apparent.

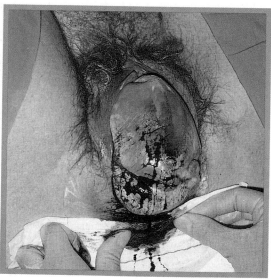

← 6.17 Breech delivery: delivery of the buttocks

The buttocks are expelled by voluntary maternal effort.

→ 6.18 Breech delivery: sacral rotation

The fetal sacrum rotates anteriorly.

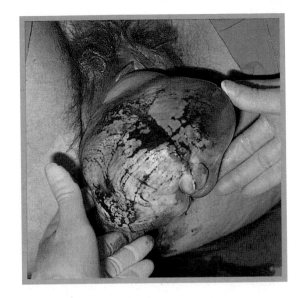

→ 6.19 Breech delivery: delivery of the legs

The legs are delivered by flexion of the thighs and knees.

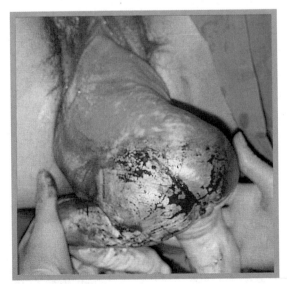

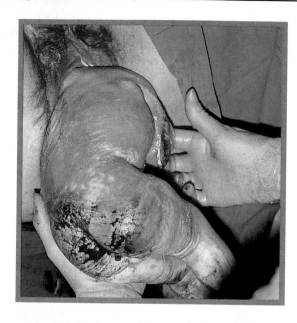

← 6.20 Breech delivery: delivery of the anterior shoulder

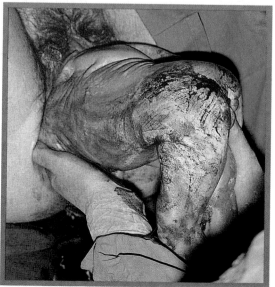

← 6.21 Breech delivery: delivery of the posterior shoulder

→ 6.22 Breech delivery: descent of the head

The trunk is allowed to hang to encourage descent of the head.

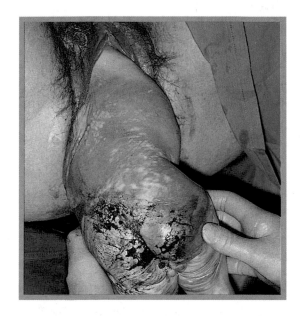

→ 6.23 Breech delivery: insertion of the first forceps blade

The trunk of the baby is swung anteriorly and the first forceps blade is inserted.

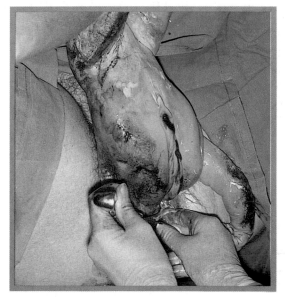

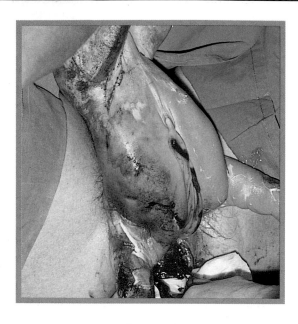

← 6.24 Breech delivery: insertion of the second forceps blade

The second blade is applied and locked into position.

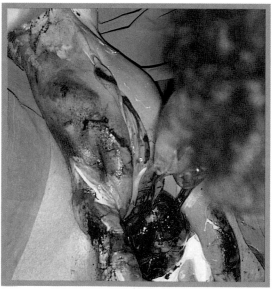

← 6.25 Breech delivery: delivery of the head

Gentle traction is applied to complete a controlled delivery of the head.

→ 6.26 Breech delivery: the third stage of labour

The third stage is completed by cord traction.

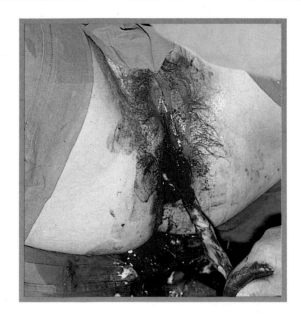

Repair of the episiotomy

Repair of the episiotomy (**6.27–6.32**) is achieved by closure of the vaginal wall, interrupted sutures into the levatores ani, and interrupted sutures to the skin.

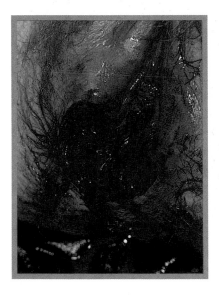

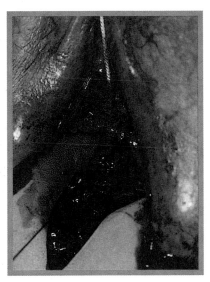

↑ 6.27 Inspection of the episiotomy

The extent of the wound is assessed.

↑ 6.28 Closure of the episiotomy

Care is taken to expose the apex of the incision in the vaginal wall and a continuous absorbable suture is used to close the vaginal wall.

→ 6.29 Closure of the episiotomy

The wound is closed to the introitus.

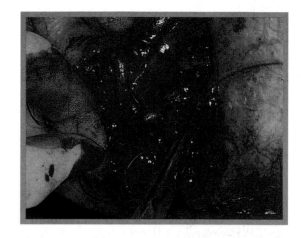

→ 6.30 Closure of the episiotomy

Care is taken to ensure that the introitus is not constricted.

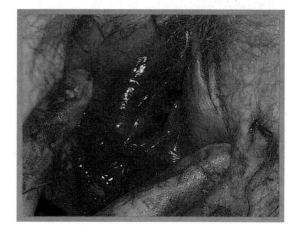

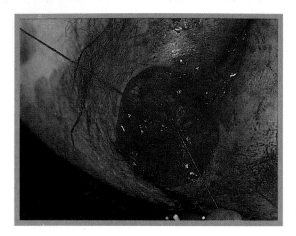

← 6.31 Closure of the episiotomy

Interrupted absorbable sutures are inserted into the levatores ani.

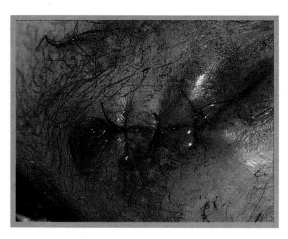

← 6.32 Closure of the episiotomy

Interrupted mattress sutures are used to close the skin.

7 Operative deliveries

Caesarean section

Caesarean section is the most widely used form of operative delivery. The incidence of operative delivery varies considerably between various countries with an incidence of 12% in the UK and figures in excess of 20% in the USA. The common indications include:
- Fetal distress.
- Cephalopelvic disproportion.
- Placenta praevia.
- Severe pre-eclampsia.

The increased incidence of Caesarean section is partly related to the desire to reduce fetal loss and partly to the greater safety of the procedure under modern conditions. (**7.1–7.24**)

Until the 1940s the common procedure was an upper segment Caesarean section, but this operation was largely abandoned because of the increased risk of uterine scar rupture during the third trimester of pregnancy. Furthermore, the postoperative complications are worse because of the increased risk of paralytic ileus, wound infection, and postpartum haemorrhage.

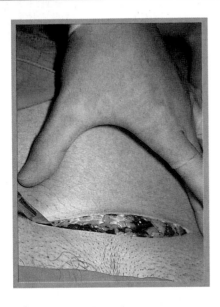

← 7.1 Caesarean section: incision

Delivery is effected through a low transverse abdominal incision.

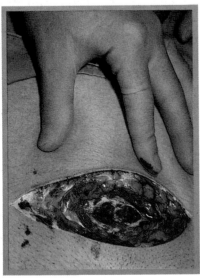

← 7.2 Caesarean section: incision

The rectus sheath is incised.

→ 7.3 Caesarean section: incision

The rectus sheath is then dissected and cut free of the rectus muscle.

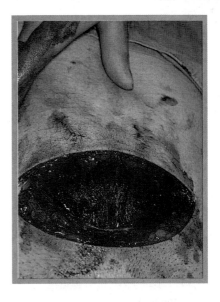

→ 7.4 Caesarean section: incision

The parietal peritoneum is incised and the abdominal cavity is opened.

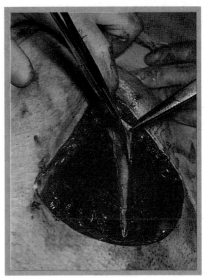

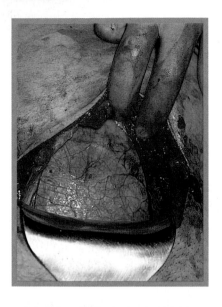

← 7.5 Caesarean section: incision

The lower uterine segment is exposed.

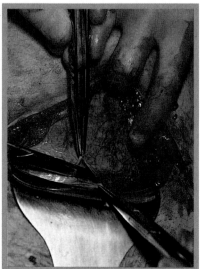

← 7.6 Caesarean section: incision

The peritoneum over the lower segment is incised.

→ 7.7 Caesarean section: incision

The peritoneum is reflected from the lower segment.

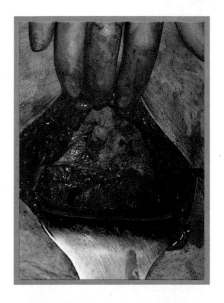

→ 7.8 Caesarean section: incision

The uterus is incised transversely and the membranes are exposed.

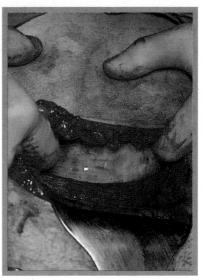

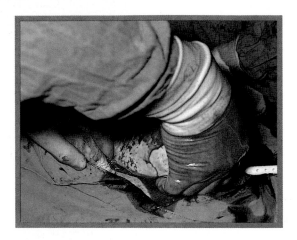

← 7.9 Caesarean section: delivery

The amniotic fluid can be seen gushing from the amniotic sac.

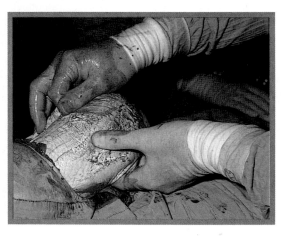

← 7.10 Caesarean section: delivery

A hand is inserted into the uterus to lift out the presenting part.

→ 7.11 Caesarean section: delivery

The presenting part—in this case the breech—is delivered by gentle traction.

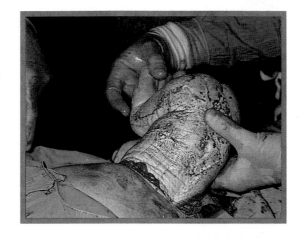

→ 7.12 Caesarean section: delivery

The legs are released and the rest of the trunk is delivered to the shoulders.

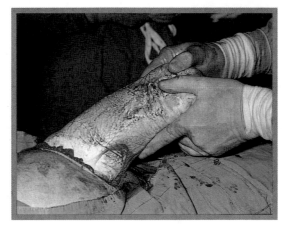

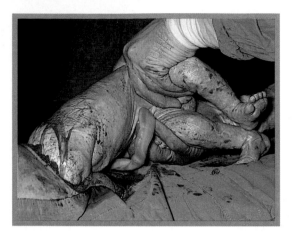

←7.13 Caesarean section: delivery

The shoulders are released by applying torsion to the trunk.

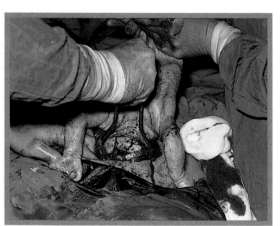

←7.14 Caesarean section: delivery

Delivery is completed by applying forceps to the head.

→ 7.15 Caesarean section: delivery

The head is released with gentle traction.

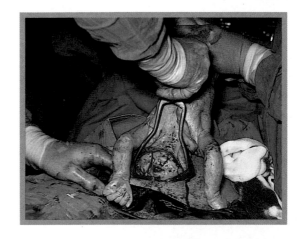

→ 7.16 Caesarean section: placental delivery

The infant is laid on the maternal abdomen, the cord is clamped, and the placenta expelled.

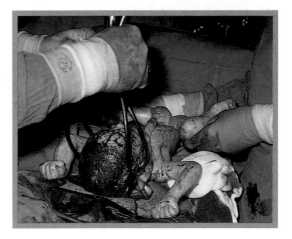

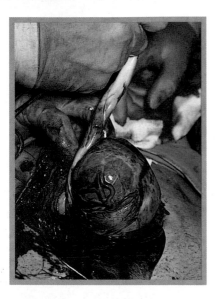

← 7.17 Caesarean section: placental delivery

The placenta is expelled through the abdominal wound.

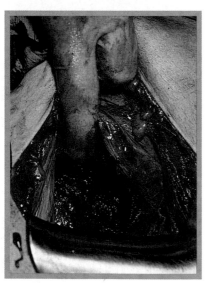

← 7.18 Caesarean section: placental delivery

The uterine cavity is explored to ensure that no placental tissue or fetal membranes are left behind.

→ 7.19 Caesarean section: closure

The edges of the uterine incision are grasped with haemostatic clamps.

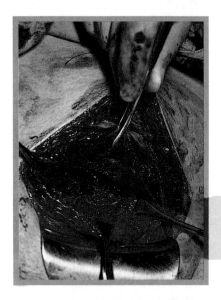

→ 7.20 Caesarean section: closure

The first layer of myometrium is closed with a continuous suture.

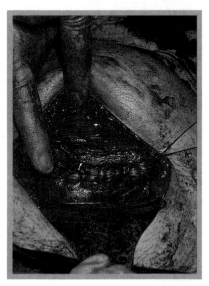

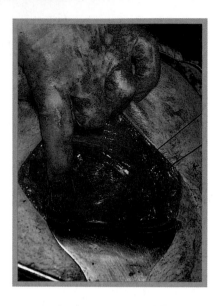

← 7.21 Caesarean section: closure

The second and outer layer is sutured.

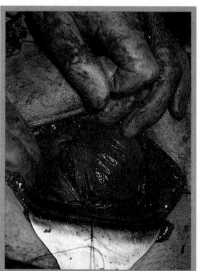

← 7.22 Caesarean section: closure

Closure of visceral peritoneum.

→ 7.23 Caesarean section: closure

Closure of the rectus sheath.

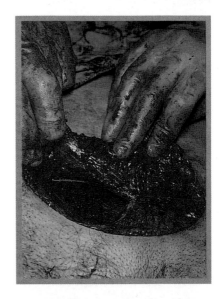

→ 7.24 Caesarean section: closure

Closure of the skin wound.

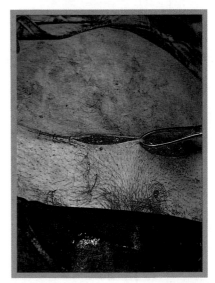

Epidural anaesthesia

Lumbar epidural anaesthesia (**7.25–7.29**) is one of the most widely used methods of pain relief in labour. It is now commonly used as a method of regional anaesthesia for Caesarean section.

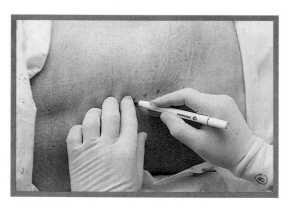

← 7.25 Epidural anaesthesia

The patient is placed on her left side with her thighs and trunk flexed. The position of the spines of the lumbar vertebrae are marked.

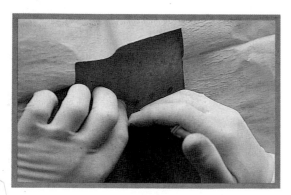

← 7.26 Epidural anaesthesia

The epidural needle is inserted between the vertebral spines of L_3 and L_4 after infiltration of the skin with local anaesthesia.

→ 7.27 Epidural anaesthesia

The resistance to the injection of a small amount of air is felt to make sure that the tip of the needle is in the epidural space.

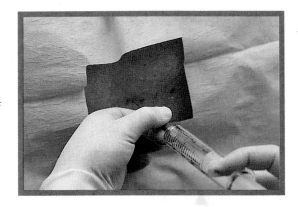

→ 7.28 Epidural anaesthesia

The epidural catheter is inserted through the needle and the needle is then removed.

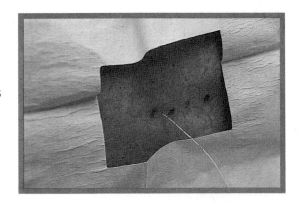

→ 7.29 Epidural anaesthesia

Epidural 'top ups' are performed by injecting local anaesthesia through a self-sealing valve.

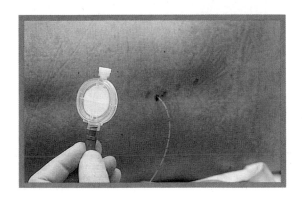

Low forceps delivery

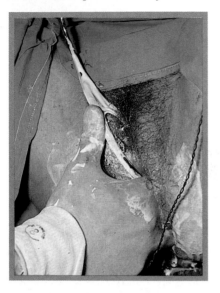

← 7.30 Low forceps delivery: insertion of the left blade

The left blade of the forceps is inserted and directly applied alongside the head.

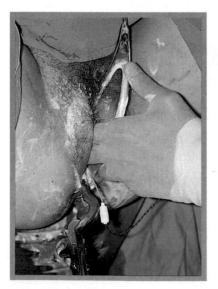

← 7.31 Low forceps delivery: application of the right blade

The right blade of the forceps is now applied to the right side of the pelvis until it lies easily alongside the fetal head.

→ 7.32 Low forceps delivery: locking the blades

The blades are now locked together.

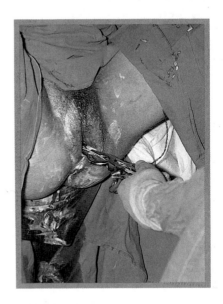

→ 7.33 Low forceps delivery: episiotomy

With the perineum stretched, a mediolateral episiotomy is cut.

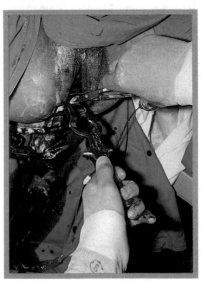

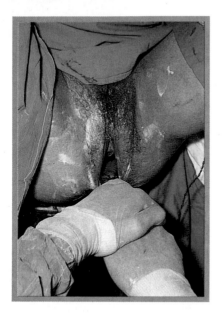

← 7.34 Low forceps delivery: descent

Traction is applied downwards and backwards to release the occiput under the pubic arch.

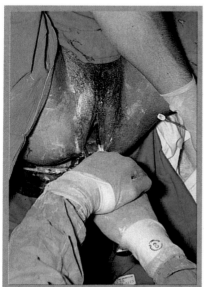

← 7.35 Low forceps delivery: descent

Further intermittent traction is applied.

→ 7.36 Low forceps delivery: descent

The scalp can now be clearly seen through the distended vulva.

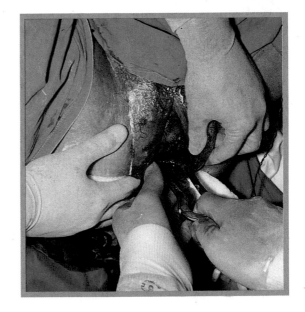

→ 7.37 Low forceps delivery: crowning of the head

The head is now beginning to crown.

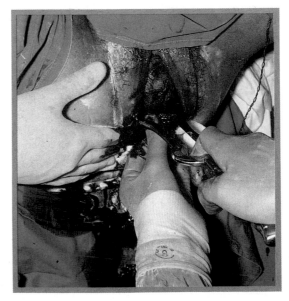

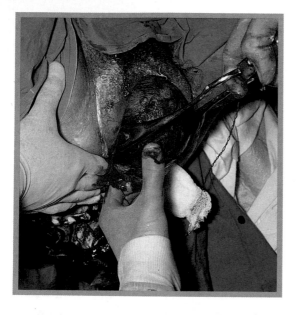

← 7.38 Low forceps delivery: crowning of the head

Maximum distension of the vulva and perineum occurs.

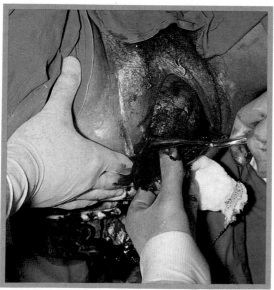

← 7.39 Low forceps delivery: delivery

As the head is delivered, the forceps blades are removed.

→ 7.40 Low forceps delivery: delivery

The umbilical cord is around the neck and is loosened before the shoulders are delivered.

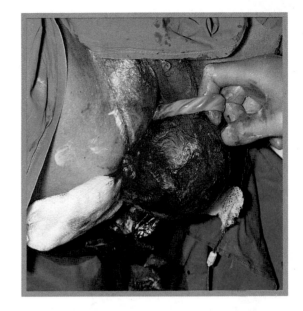

→ 7.41 Low forceps delivery: delivery

The anterior shoulder is delivered by downward traction on the head.

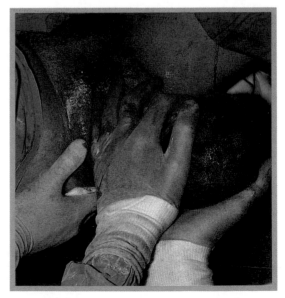

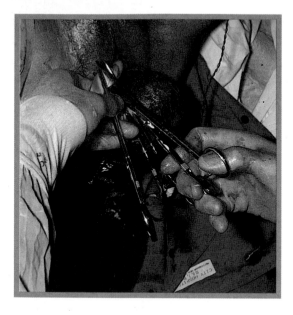

← 7.42 Low forceps delivery: delivery

The umbilical cord is cut and clamped.

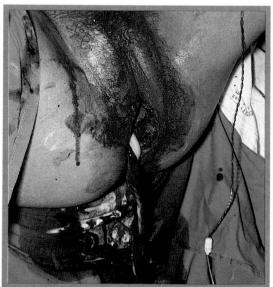

← 7.43 Low forceps delivery: delivery

Delivery of the child is complete. The placenta is still in the uterus.

→ 7.44 Low forceps delivery: placental delivery

After checking that the uterus is firmly contracted, cord traction is applied with suprapubic pressure on the uterus.

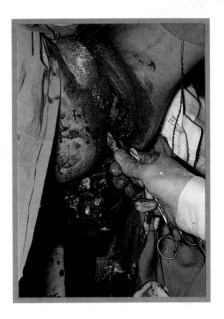

→ 7.45 Low forceps delivery: placental delivery

The placenta descends into the vagina.

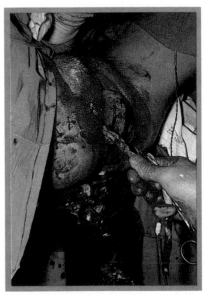

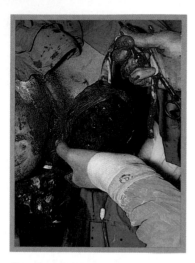

↑ 7.46 Low forceps delivery: placental delivery

The placental expulsion is complete and the placenta and membranes are examined.

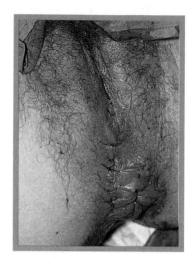

↑ 7.47 Low forceps delivery: repair of episiotomy

The episiotomy is sutured.

8 | Ultrasound

and magnetic

resonance imaging

The introduction of ultrasound in imaging of the female pelvis and the fetus has revolutionised the management of abnormalities in pregnancy and the diagnosis of gynaecological pathology. The images produced in this section are no more than samples to illustrate the value of these techniques in some areas of clinical practice.

Ultrasound imaging

Ultrasound imaging is based on the direction of sound waves with frequencies between 2–20 megahertz into the tissues of the pelvis and abdominal cavity. The returning echoes from tissue interfaces of differing densities are used to construct images of the target site. Ultrasound is produced by the excitation of the piezo-electric crystal. The transmission phase is short and the 'transmitting' crystal reverts to a receiving phase.

Most modern instruments are real-time scanners and are available in three forms.
• Linear array.
• Mechanical array.
• Phased array.
The quality of images continues to improve. However, ultrasound imaging is always limited to demonstrating physical structure (**8.1–8.37**) and not biochemical composition.

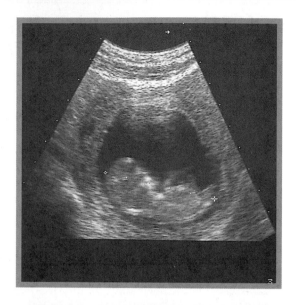

←8.1 Crown–rump length

The measurement of crown–rump length is demonstrated in this picture and is the technique used in early pregnancy to assess gestational age.

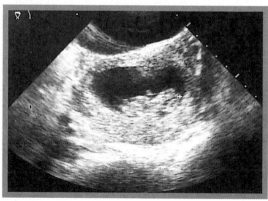

←8.2 Crown–rump length

A crown–rump length of 40 mm is demonstrated in this film in early pregnancy.

→ 8.3 At 13 weeks' gestation

The whole fetus demonstrated in longitudinal section.

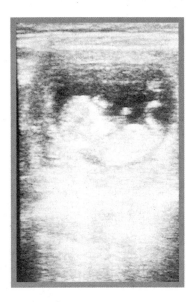

→ 8.4 At 14 weeks' gestation

The features of the face can now be seen.

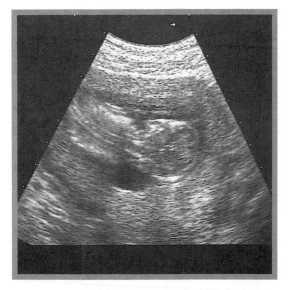

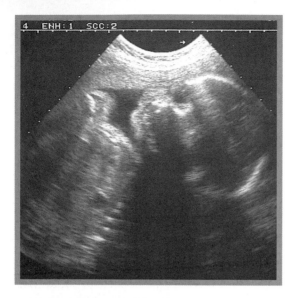

← 8.5 Facial structure

The details of facial structure can be seen with remarkable clarity.

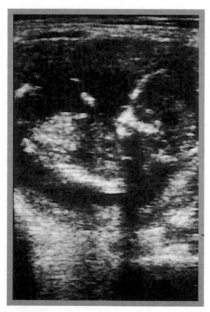

← 8.6 At 15 weeks' gestation

A normal fetus.

→ 8.7 Fetal spine

The fetal spine can be screened in sufficient detail to allow recognition of spina bifida and is used as a screening procedure.

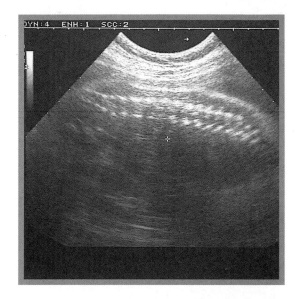

→ 8.8 A male fetus identified by the external genitalia

This is not always possible and the identification of the sex of the fetus is therefore not always reliable.

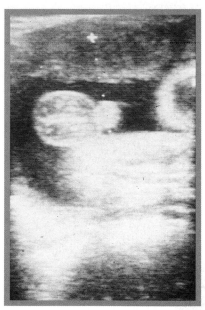

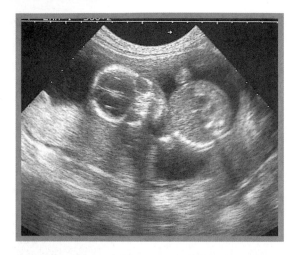

← 8.9 At 18 weeks' gestation

At this time the structures of all organs are screened.

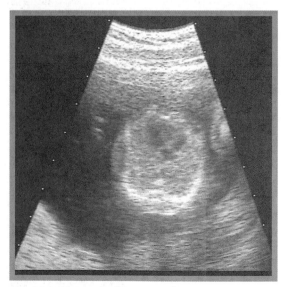

← 8.10 Fetal heart

Imaging of the four chambers of the fetal heart.

→ 8.11 Fetal heart

A further four-chamber view of the fetal heart showing the foramen ovale.

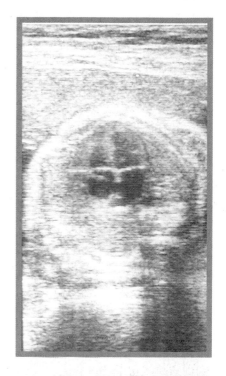

→ 8.12 Measurement of head circumference

This allows an assessment of fetal growth and gestational age.

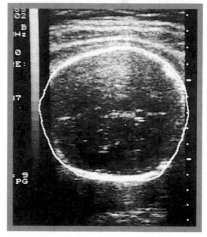

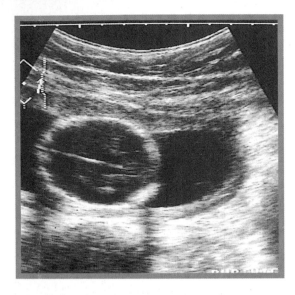

← 8.13
Measurement of head circumference

If the section is too high, assessment of gestational age can be inaccurate.

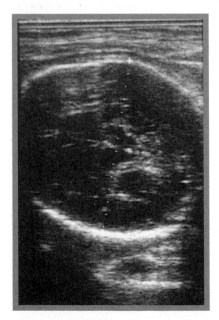

← 8.14 Measurement of biparietal diameter

This was the earliest method of assessing gestational age. The diameter in this picture is 82 mm.

→ 8.15 Cerebral ventricles

Demonstration of the cerebral ventricles in a normal fetus.

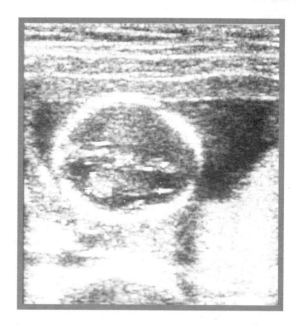

→ 8.16 Measurement of abdominal circumference

This is valuable in the assessment of asymmetrical growth retardation.

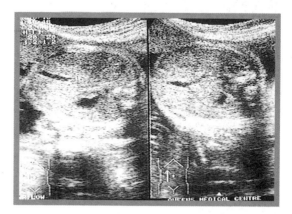

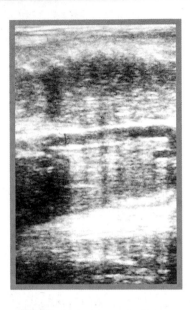

← 8.17 Doppler blood velocity measurement

The fetal aorta is visible in this film and is used for Doppler blood velocity measurement.

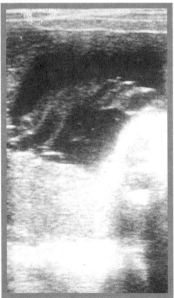

← 8.18 Umbilical cord

The structure and position of the umbilical cord are seen and can be used for obtaining blood samples from the fetus.

→ 8.19 Twin pregnancy

The early detection of a twin
pregnancy has been particularly
useful in the management of
multiple pregnancies.

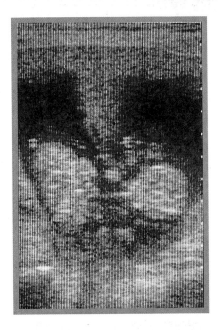

→ 8.20 Amniocentesis

This is commonly performed at 16
weeks' gestation. The needle can be
seen on this film.

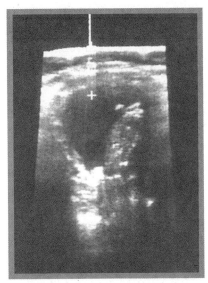

Congenital abnormalities: ultrasound images

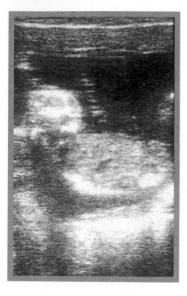

← 8.21 Anencephaly

The cranial vault is missing.

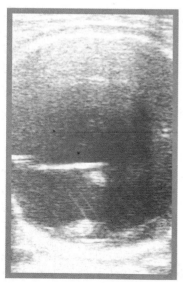

← 8.22 Hydrocephalus associated with spina bifida

→ 8.23 Spina bifida

Transverse section.

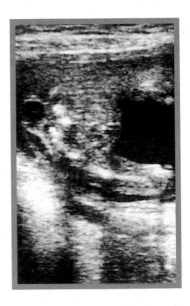

→ 8.24 Holoprosencephaly

This condition is associated with a fluid-filled cranial vault, a small skull, disorganised cerebral ventricles, and prominent basal nuclei.

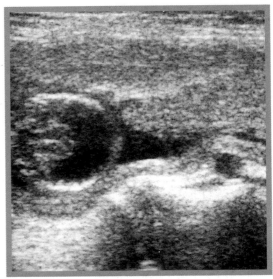

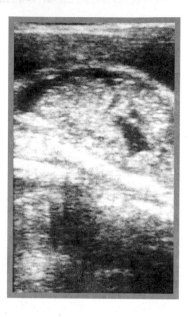

← 8.25 Fetal ascites

Fetal ascites with fluid distension of the abdominal cavity.

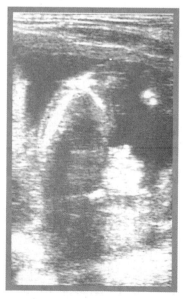

← 8.26 Gastroschisis

Gastroschisis with extrusion of the fetal bowel.

→ 8.27 Exomphalos

This defect in the abdominal wall is more severe and the eviscerated organs include small intestine and liver.

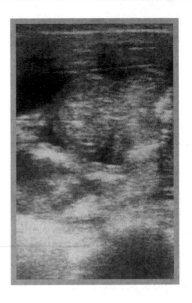

Gynaecological conditions: ultrasound images

→ 8.28 Hydatidiform mole

This shows the mottled snow storm appearance of the molar tissue.

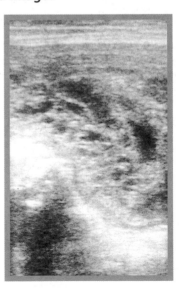

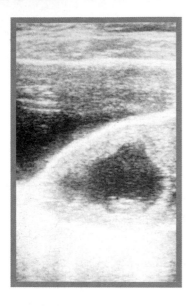

← 8.29 Missed abortion

The conceptus is small and lies inside a disproportionately large sac. The size of the conceptus is not consistent with the gestational age and a fetal heart beat cannot be detected.

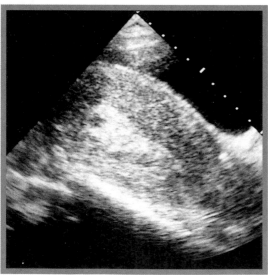

← 8.30 Retained products of conception

Placental tissue can be seen in the uterine cavity.

→ 8.31 Normal endometrium

The thickness of normal endometrium can be measured with ultrasound.

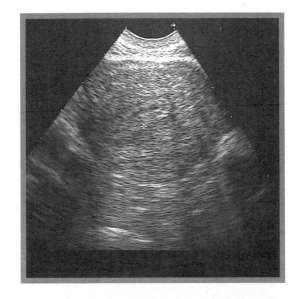

→ 8.32 Lippes loop

Location of a Lippes loop inside the uterine cavity.

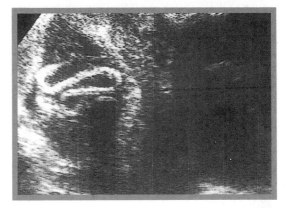

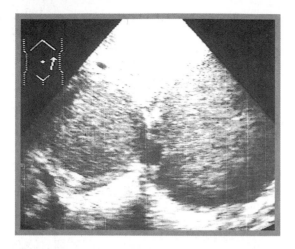

← 8.33 Two endometriotic (chocolate) cysts

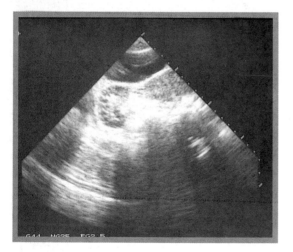

← 8.34 Polycystic ovaries

Ultrasound scanning of the pelvis provides the simplest method of diagnosing polycystic ovaries. Multiple small cysts can be seen throughout the ovarian cortex.

→ 8.35 Multiple large ovarian cysts

Grossly hyperstimulated ovaries showing multiple large ovarian cysts.

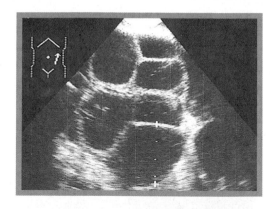

→ 8.36 A solitary, simple ovarian cyst

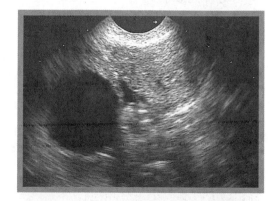

→ 8.37 A solitary, intramural uterine fibroid

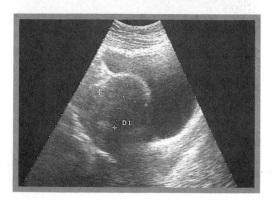

Magnetic resonance imaging

The use of magnetic resonance imaging (MRI) has been limited in obstetrics, but is more widespread in gynaecology (**8.38–8.44**). It depends on the use of powerful magnetic fields and pulsed radio frequencies to create maps of proton densities that give a high quality image of physical structure. With the use of spectroscopy, it can also be used to image biochemical reactions, but this has not been fully exploited in clinical imaging in obstetrics and gynaecology.

Fetus and placenta: magnetic resonance images

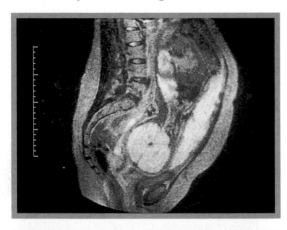

← 8.38 A normal fetus (sagittal view) at 36 weeks' gestation

This shows the fetal brain, the placenta, and fetal lung using a T2-weighted sequence.

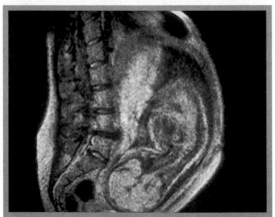

← 8.39 A posterior, low-lying placenta

The internal cervical os can be clearly visualised, allowing precise placental localisation.

→ 8.40 Umbilical cord at the abdominal insertion

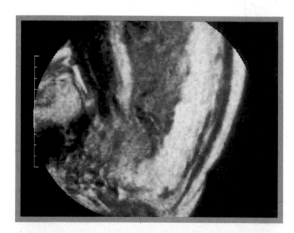

→ 8.41 Buccal fat in a full term fetus

T1-weighted sequence highlighting the buccal fat in a full term fetus.

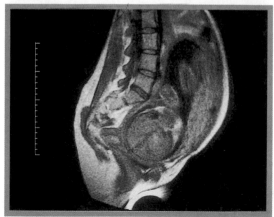

Gynaecology: magnetic resonance images

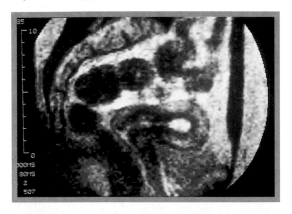

← 8.42 A normal pelvis

This demonstrates the harsh white appearance of the endometrium, the non-resonant subendometrial zone, and the clear outline of the myometrium.

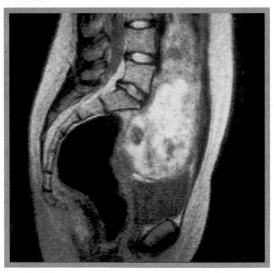

← 8.43 Hydatidiform mole

Molar tissue can be seen invading the uterine wall.

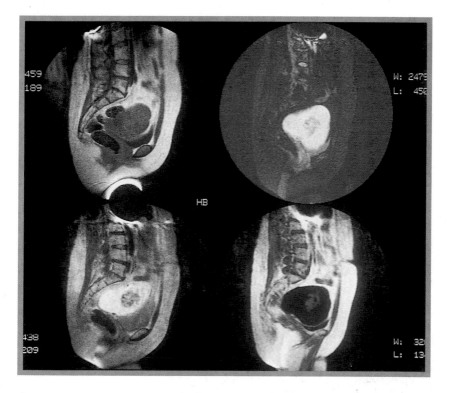

↑ 8.44 Ovarian carcinoma

Different imaging sequences of an ovarian carcinoma. These highlight the interval structure of the tumour. Top left T_1/T_2; top right STIR sequence; bottom left T_2; bottom right T_1.

9 | Gynaecology

Understanding the anatomy (**9.1–9.16**) and histology (**9.17–9.23**) of the pelvic organs is fundamental to understanding the range and effects of pelvic pathology. The relationship of the major organs within the pelvic cavity determines the course of malignant disease of the cervix and corpus uteri. Furthermore, understanding the processes involved in fertilisation and implantation depends on an appreciation of the cyclical changes in the endometrium and their relationship to the corresponding hormonal changes in the healthy sexually mature female.

The pathology of the pelvis and the female pelvic organs is extensive and varied. The ovary produces tumours of remarkable complexity and variability because it is totipotential. This book shows examples of the wide range of conditions, both congenital and acquired, encountered in the practice of gynaecology.

Anatomy of the pelvic organs

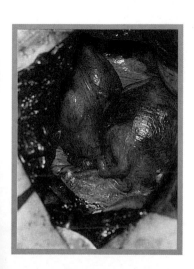

← 9.1 Looking into the pelvis at the time of hysterectomy

The fundus of the uterus can be seen with the right fallopian tube emerging from the uterine fundus.

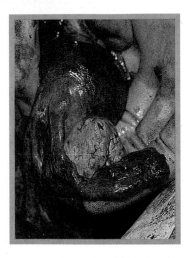

← 9.2 Looking into the pelvis at the time of hysterectomy

The left tube and ovary can be seen lying on the posterior leaf of the broad ligament.

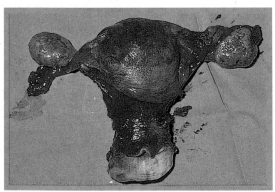

← 9.3 The uterus, tubes, and ovaries

Removed at the time of pelvic clearance.

→ 9.4 Gross hemisection of the pelvis

This shows the midline viscera and structures on the pelvic side wall. The dissection shows the obturator artery, vein, and nerve. In addition, the uterine artery and ureter, umbilical artery, ovary, and broad ligament can be seen.

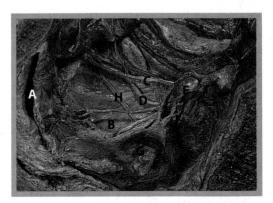

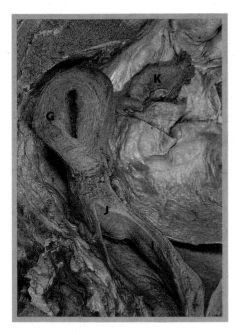

A	Bladder
B	Ureter
C	Obturator nerve
D	Obturator artery
E	Ovary
F	Broad ligament
G	Uterus
H	Obturator vein
I	Vagina
J	Cervix
K	Uterine tube
L	Rectum
M	Intestine
N	Anal canal
O	Symphysis
P	Ischiocavernosus
Q	Bulbospongiosus
R	Small intestine
S	Venous plexus
T	Levator ani
U	Ischial ramus
V	Obturator internus
W	Superior pubic ramus
X	Pubis
Y	Promontory of sacrum
Z	Cauda equina

↑ 9.5 Uterus, vagina and cervix

Close-up view of a dissection showing the cervix protruding into the vaginal vault.

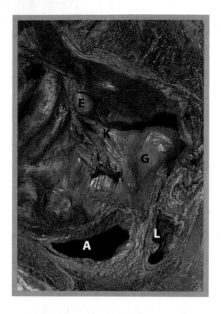

← 9.6 Hemisection of the pelvis

This shows mid-line viscera, bladder, rectum, uterus, broad ligament, and ovary. Side wall left undissected, but external iliac vessels visible at pelvic brim.

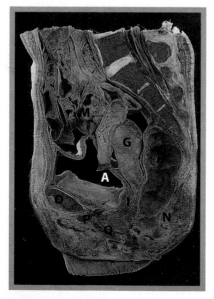

← 9.7 Sagittal section through the pelvis

This shows coils of gut, bladder, uterus, vagina, rectum, anal canal, ischiocavernosus, and bulbospongiosis muscles.

→ 9.8 The opposite side of 9.7

Gluteus maximus, a plexus of vessels around the vagina, levator ani muscle, obturator internus muscle, bladder, gut, and uterus can be identified.

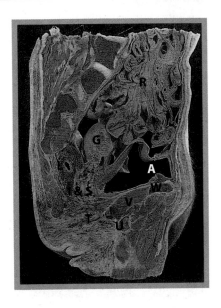

A	Bladder
B	Ureter
C	Obturator nerve
D	Obturator artery
E	Ovary
F	Broad ligament
G	Uterus
H	Obturator vein
I	Vagina
J	Cervix
K	Uterine tube
L	Rectum
M	Intestine
N	Anal canal
O	Symphysis
P	Ischiocavernosus
Q	Bulbospongiosus
R	Small intestine
S	Venous plexus
T	Levator ani
U	Ischial ramus
V	Obturator internus
W	Superior pubic ramus
X	Pubis
Y	Promontory of sacrum
Z	Cauda equina

→ 9.9 A parasagittal section

This shows similar features to 9.8.

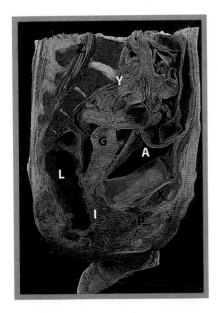

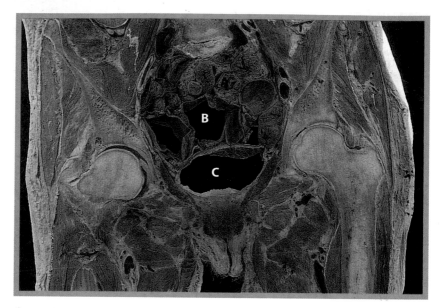

↑ 9.10 Vertical section through the pelvis in a coronal plane

The hip joints and surrounding muscles can be seen, as well as the bladder, levator ani muscle, and coils of intestine.

A	Small intestine	O	Rectum
B	Sigmoid colon	P	External iliac arteryand vein
C	Bladder	Q	Roof of acetabulum
D	Gluteal muscles	R	Rectal ampulla
E	Coils of small intestine	S	Femoral artery and vein
F	Trigone	T	Obturator neurovascular
G	Obturator internus		bundle
H	Obturator externus	U	Urethra
I	Levator ani	V	Vagina
J	Sacrum	W	Ischiorectal fossa
K	Piriformis	X	Anal canal
L	Broad ligament	Y	Gluteus maximus
M	Uterus	Z	Clitoris
N	Symphysis		

Gynaecology

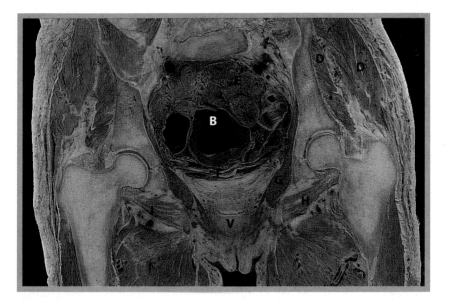

↑ 9.11 Vertical section in a coronal plane

This shows the vagina as well as a profile of the bladder trigone with the ureteric orifices.

→ 9.12 Horizontal section through the pelvis

This shows sacrum piriformis muscle, rectum, uterus, coils of gut, and gluteus maximus and medius muscles.

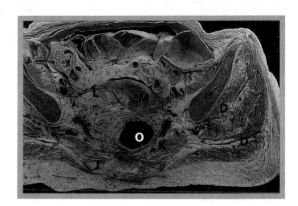

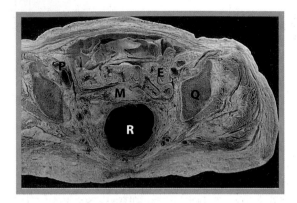

← 9.13 Section
taken 2 cm below
9.12

← 9.13 Section taken 2 cm below 9.12

This shows the rectal ampulla, uterus, ureter, coils of gut, external iliac vessels, and the coccyx.

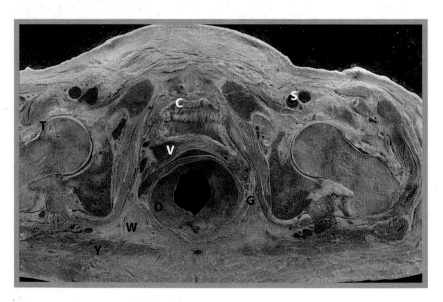

↑ 9.14 Section taken 4 cm below 9.13

The rectal ampulla, vagina, and bladder can be seen, as well as the obturator internus muscle, gluteus maximus muscle, the inferior vessels, the ischiorectal fossa, and the hip joints.

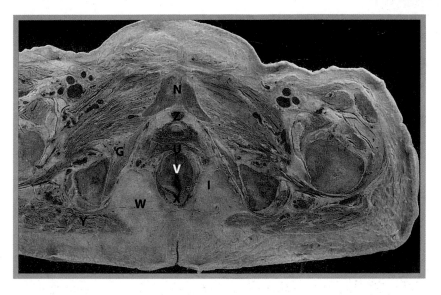

↑ 9.15 Section taken 2 cm below 9.14

This shows the anal canal, ischiorectal fossa, vagina, urethra, obturator internus muscle, levator ani muscle, and clitoris.

A	Small intestine	O	Rectum
B	Sigmoid colon	P	External iliac arteryand vein
C	Bladder	Q	Roof of acetabulum
D	Gluteal muscles	R	Rectal ampulla
E	Coils of small intestine	S	Femoral artery and vein
F	Trigone	T	Obturator neurovascular bundle
G	Obturator internus		
H	Obturator externus	U	Urethra
I	Levator ani	V	Vagina
J	Sacrum	W	Ischiorectal fossa
K	Piriformis	X	Anal canal
L	Broad ligament	Y	Gluteus maximus
M	Uterus	Z	Clitoris
N	Symphysis		

Histology of the endometrium

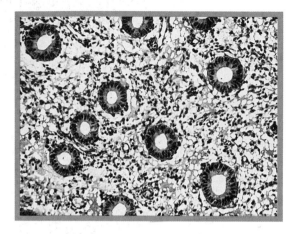

← 9.16 Proliferative phase of the endometrium

The surface epithelium is low and cuboidal. The glands are straight with no tendency to convolution. The stroma appears dense, compact, and non-vascular.

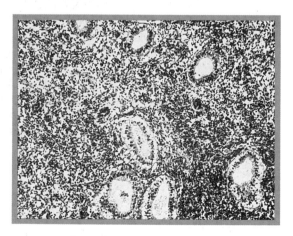

← 9.17 Early secretory phase endometrium

The surface epithelium is taller and definitely columnar and the glands become hypertrophic and convoluted, with evidence of secretory activity.

→ 9.18 Mid-secretory phase

The secretory activity of the epithelium becomes increasingly marked, with glycogen granules in the epithelium and sometimes in the lumina of the glands.

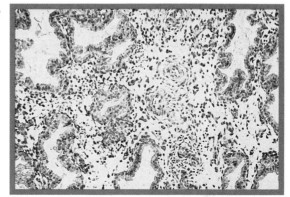

→ 9.19 Late secretory phase endometrium

This shows glandular as well as stromal changes. The saw-tooth pattern is characteristic and there is stromal invasion by 'pseudo-inflammatory cells'.

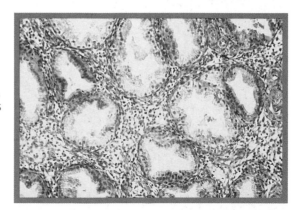

→ 9.20 Menstrual endometrium

There is marked cellular infiltration of the upper layer, accompanied by small haematomas and surface tissue loss.

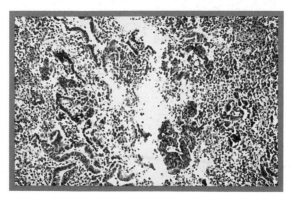

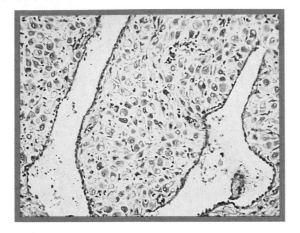

←9.21 Decidualised endometrium

Stromal cells become large and polygonal with a wide zone of cytoplasm surrounding the nucleus. The decidual cells are arranged in a mosaic or tile-like fashion.

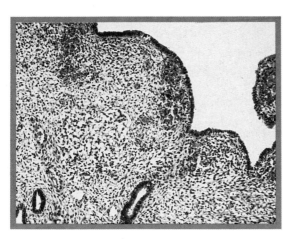

←9.22 'Pill effect'

This shows the paucity of glandular activity and the decidual appearance of the stroma.

10 Lesions of the vulva and vagina

Examination of the vulva is an integral and important part of every gynaecological examination. The appearance of the vulva and vagina varies normally in relation to age and hormone status and changes in the skin of the vulva and vagina must take into account the expected texture of the epithelium for any given age. Good lighting and, where indicated, a magnifying glass or a colposcope, are needed for a systematic examination.

Both benign and malignant tumours of the vulva and vagina are relatively uncommon.

Congenital abnormalities of the vagina

The simplest vaginal abnormality which is easily treated by incision is the imperforate hymen (**10.1**). Congenital absence of the vagina results from defective formation of the müllerian ducts, and can be remedied by creating a space between the bladder and rectum, and inserting a mould covered by amnion or skin (**10.2–10.7**). The uterus is sometimes present, but has no external vaginal passage. Under these circumstances, a vagina must be created and the uterus connected to this cavity (**10.8–10.14**).

Congenital septum of the vagina can be easily divided, but is often asymptomatic (**10.15**).

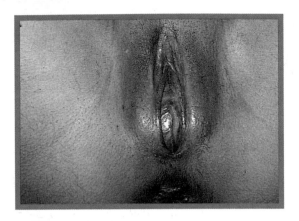

↑ 10.1 Imperforate hymen

Menstrual loss has accumulated in the vagina and can be seen bulging the hymen.

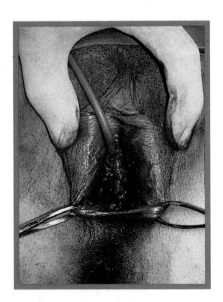

← 10.2 Vaginal agenesis

The indentation over the normal site of the vaginal introitus can be seen. The uterus was absent in this patient, but the ovaries were present and the development of secondary sexual characteristics was normal.

→ 10.3 Vaginal agenesis: surgery

Creation of a canal between the bladder and rectum allows the insertion of a mould in order to create an artificial vagina.

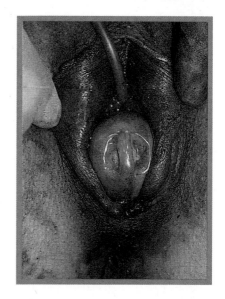

→ 10.4 Vaginal agenesis: surgery

The remnants of the müllerian ducts may be demonstrated after reflection of the surface epithelium.

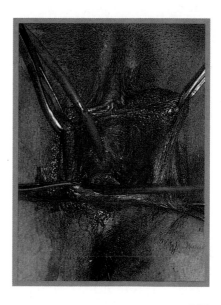

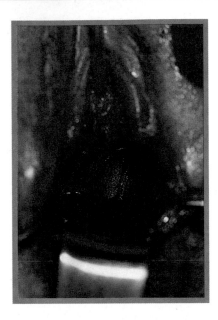

← 10.5 Vaginal agenesis: surgery

A space is created between the
bladder and rectum.

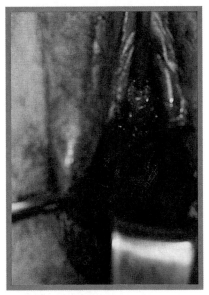

← 10.6 Vaginal agenesis: surgery

It is important to achieve haemostasis if
the amnion graft is to be retained.

→ 10.7 Vaginal agenesis: surgery

An inflatable plastic mould is sutured into the vagina and held in place by labial closure. The mould can be reinflated by injecting fluid into the reservoir.

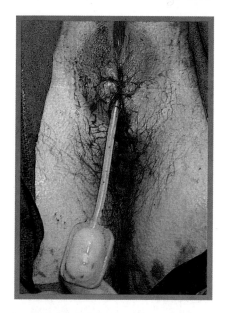

→ 10.8 Vaginal agenesis

This woman presented with pain every month and was subsequently shown to have uterine tissue with a haematometra.

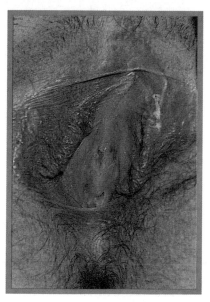

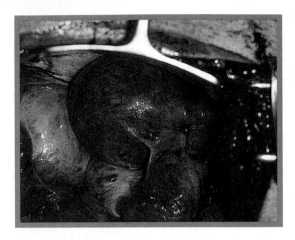

← 10.9 Vaginal agenesis

The uterus is distended and retrograde spill of menstrual loss had led to the development of endometriotic patches.

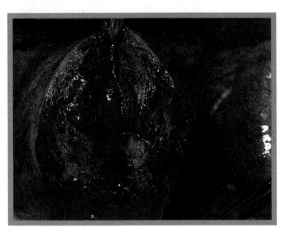

← 10.10 Vaginal agenesis

The uterine cavity is opened. It contains old, altered menstrual loss.

→ 10.11 Vaginal agenesis: surgery

A catheter is inserted into the uterine cavity to connect it with the vaginal cavity.

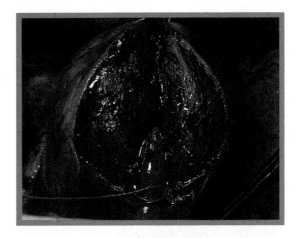

→ 10.12 Vaginal agenesis: surgery

Closure of the uterine incision after insertion of the uterine catheter.

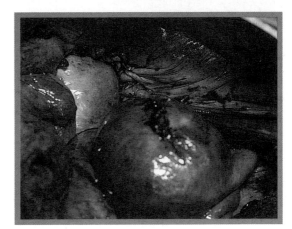

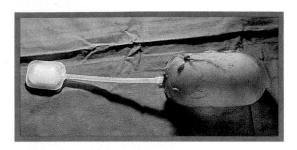

← 10.13 Vaginal agenesis: surgery

An inflatable vaginal mould is inserted into the vaginal space.

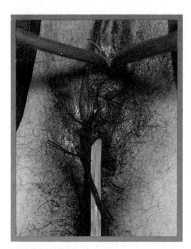

← 10.14 Vaginal agenesis: surgery

Two catheters—one from the uterine cavity and one from the vaginal space—are shown draining the vulval wound.

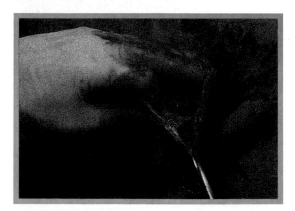

← 10.15 Congenital septum of the vagina

This can be easily divided. The patient may present with dyspareunia or postcoital bleeding, but is often asymptomatic.

Lesions of the vulva

Various benign lesions of the vulva are demonstrated. These may be acquired or neoplastic (**10.16–10.21**), or congenital (**10.16**).

Vaginal prolapse is commonly, but not invariably, associated with uterine descent, and results in protrusion of both the anterior vaginal wall (cystocele) and posterior vaginal wall (rectocele) (**10.22–10.24**). Urethral caruncles are common (**10.25**), whereas clitoral hypertrophy (**10.26**) is relatively rare. **10.27** shows a gross example of herpetic vulvitis.

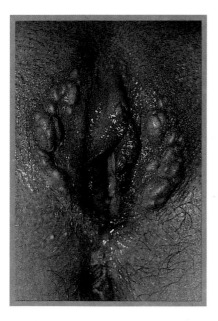

↑ **10.16 Vulval lipomas**

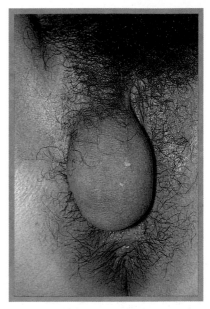

↑ **10.17 Benign vulval cyst**

A large Wolffian duct cyst arising from a vestige of the Wolffian duct.

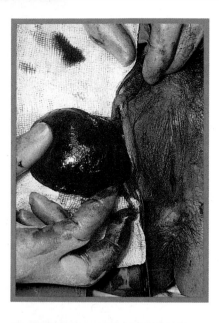

← 10.18 Benign vulval cyst: surgery

An incision is made through the labial skin to expose the cyst.

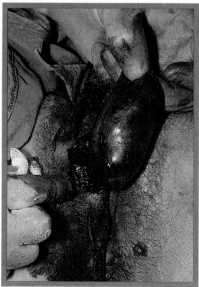

← 10.19 Benign vulval cyst: surgery

The cyst is fully exposed and dissected free from its underlying bed.

→ 10.20 Benign vulval cyst: surgery

The wound is closed after excision of the cyst.

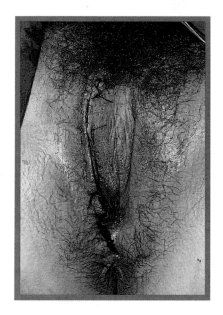

→ 10.21 Large benign cystic tumour of the vulva

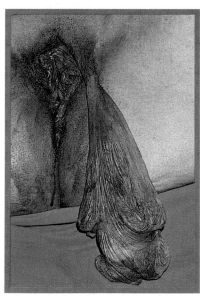

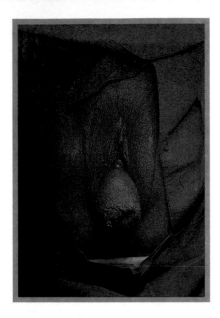

← 10.22 Procidentia

A third-degree prolapse of the uterus and vaginal walls.

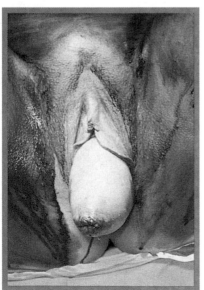

← 10.23 Procidentia with a large cystocoele

→ 10.24 Procidentia

Procidentia associated with
dependent ulceration of the vaginal
skin.

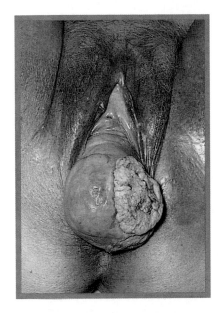

→ 10.25 Urethral caruncle

The caruncle is a reddened, tender
polypoid lesion arising from the
posterior portion of the urethral
meatus.

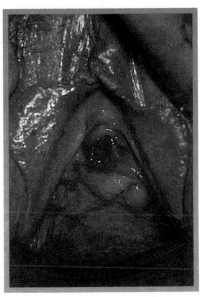

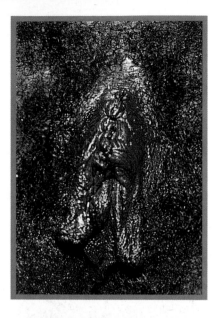

← 10.26 Clitoral enlargement

Clitoral enlargement is associated with increased androgen secretion from an arrhenoblastoma.

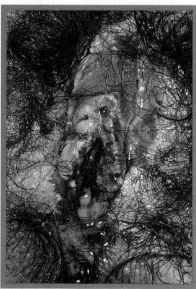

← 10.27 Herpetic vulvitis

This infection is caused by herpes simplex virus. Lesions can occur in the cervix and in the perivulvar region.

Vulvar disease

The classification of vulvar disease depends on histological examination of a skin biopsy. Classification of vulval dystrophies is now listed as shown in **Table 10.1**.

Some examples of vulval dystrophies are shown (**10.28–10.32**). The majority of vulval carcinomas are squamous cell lesions, and are generally exophytic in nature (**10.33–10.35**).

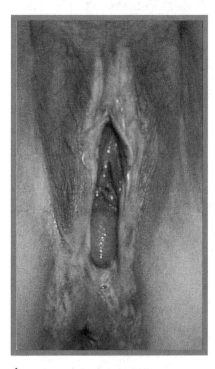

I Non-neoplastic epithelial disorders of skin and mucosa
   1 Lichen sclerosus (lichen sclerosus et atrophicus)
   2 Squamous cell hyperplasia (formerly hyperplastic dystrophy)
   3 Other dermatoses

II Vulvar intra-epithelialneoplasia (VIN)
   VINI
   Mild dysplasia (formerly mild atypia)
   VINII
   Moderate dysplasia (formerly moderate atypia)
   VINIII
   Severe dysplasia (formerly severe atypia)
   VINIV
   Carcinoma *in situ*

↑ **Table 10.1 Classification of vulval dystrophies**

↑ **10.28 Lichen sclerosus**

Histological findings are thinning of the epidermis, subepidermal hyalinisation, and the presence of a deep band of inflammatory cells.

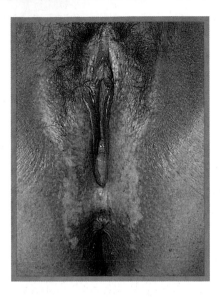

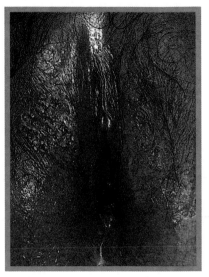

↑ 10.29 Leukoplakic vulvitis

Leukoplakic changes are associated with hyperkeratosis, irregular rete pegs, and dermal collagenisation.

↑ 10.30 Basal cell carcinoma of the vulva

This is involving the right labium majus.

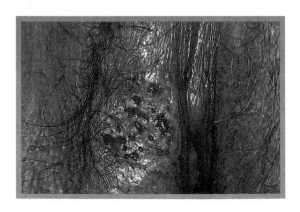

← 10.31 Basal cell carcinoma of the vulva

Close-up view.

→ 10.32 Pigmented intraepithelial neoplasia or Bowen's disease of the vulva

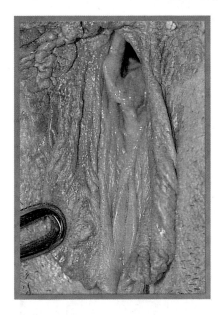

→ 10.33 Exophytic vulval carcinoma

The tumour is fungating and infected, with areas of necrosis.

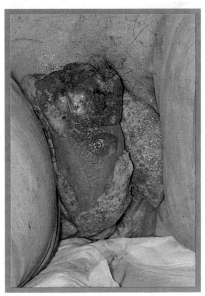

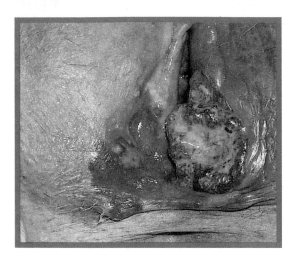

← 10.34 Ulcerative squamous cell carcinoma of the vulva

Most of these tumours are squamous cell carcinomas.

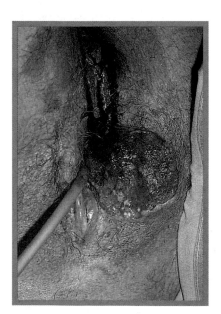

← 10.35 Fungating squamous cell carcinoma of the vulva

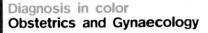
11 | The cervix

The cervix uteri is the portion of the uterus that lies below the internal cervical os. It responds to the hormonal changes of the menstrual cycle. The changes are less obvious than those seen in the endometrium, but are particularly clear during the course of pregnancy.

The epithelium of the cervix is of two types. The section that protrudes into the vagina is lined by stratified squamous epithelium. The epithelium of the endocervix is lined by a cylindrical 'picket-fence' type of endocervical epithelium. This is much taller than the epithelium of the endometrium. The nuclei of the lining cells are placed basally. The glands of the cervix are of the racemose type and this epithelium normally shows no cornification. The transition may be sudden as the external epithelium joins the squamous epithelium at the squamocolumnar junction. The glands of the cervix are lined by epithelium similar to that which lines the endocervix.

The stroma of the cervix consists primarily of connective tissue with an increasing admixture of muscle cells as it nears the internal os. During pregnancy, there is a marked increase in the actual number of glands and the glands are increased in size and tortuosity, making up half the bulk of the cervix. There is also hyperplasia of the glandular epithelium.

Decidual reaction within a mosaic pattern in the stroma of the cervix suggests the presence of stromal cells within the stroma.

Examinations of the appearances of the normal cervix and of various pathological conditions are shown (11.1–11.8). Cervical cytology is an essential component of any cervical examination; (11.19–11.22) demonstrate the microscopic appearances of the cellular components of the smear.

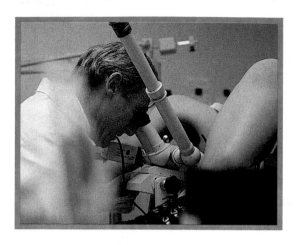

← 11.1 Examination of the cervix

This can be achieved by direct inspection or by inspection through the colposcope.

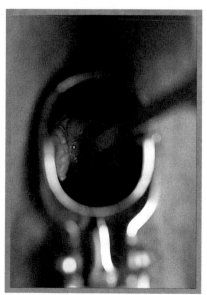

← 11.2 Cervical cytology

This forms the basis of screening programmes for carcinoma of the cervix and is a routine part of the vaginal examination.

→ 11.3 Normal multiparous cervix

The normal multiparous cervix treated with a dilute solution of acetic acid.

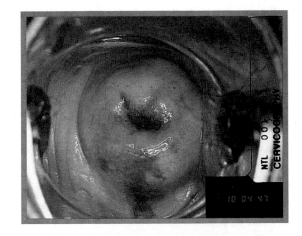

→ 11.4 Normal cervix

Stained with Schiller's iodine. The squamo-columnar junction can be seen because only normal squamous epithelium stains.

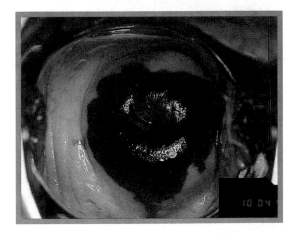

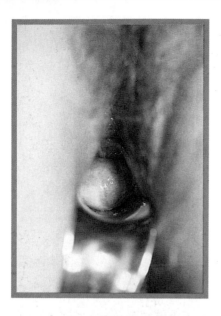

← 11.5 Fibroid polyp protruding through the external cervical os

This polyp probably arises within the uterine cavity.

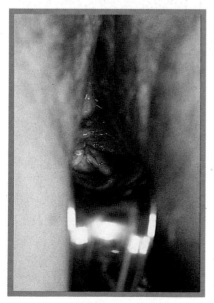

← 11.6 Small endocervical polyp

Such polyps may be lined with either squamous or columnar epithelium.

→ 11.7 Cervical intraepithelial neoplasia (CIN) stage I

Acetowhite appearance of part of the anterior lip of the cervix associated with cervical intra-epithelial neoplasia (CIN) Stage I. This relates to mild dyskaryosis in the cervical smear.

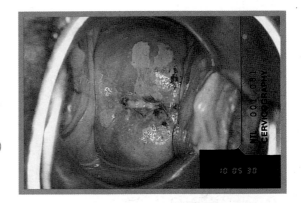

→ 11.8 CIN2

The degree of histological abnormality is reflected in the intercapillary distance

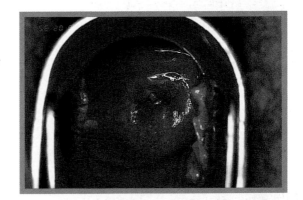

→ 11.9 CIN2

The abnormal epithelium fails to stain with iodine.

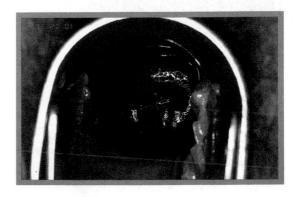

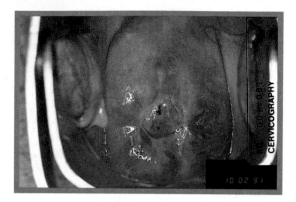

← 11.10 CIN3

The lesion is predominantly around the external os.

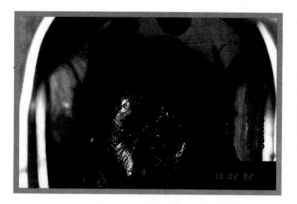

← 11.11 CIN3

Histological examination of a biopsy taken from the non-staining area shows mitotic figures scattered throughout the thickness of the epithelium with no surface stratification.

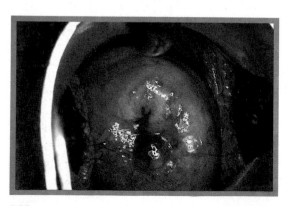

← 11.12 CIN3

A further example. It is difficult to differentiate the grading of CIN by the colposcopic appearances.

→11.13 CIN3

The non-iodine staining areas can be seen around the external os.

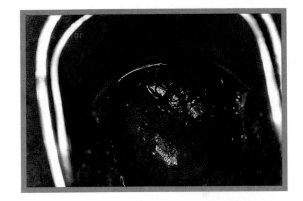

→11.14 Human papilloma virus infection

Colposcopic appearances of human papilloma virus infection before the application of acetic acid.

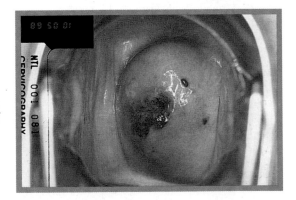

→11.15 Human papilloma virus infection

A further example of human papilloma virus infection of the cervix.

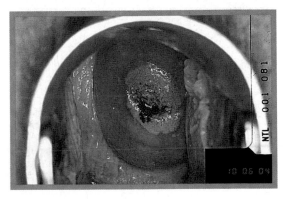

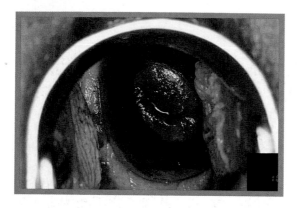

← 11.16 Human papilloma virus infection

The same cervix stained with Lugol's iodine. The limits of the abnormal epithelium are clearly demarcated.

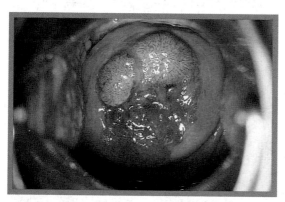

← 11.17 Cervical condylomata acuminata

These are gross lesions arising from tumour papilloma virus infection and are exophytic with multiple fine finger-like projections.

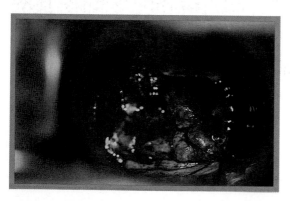

← 11.18 Exophytic invasive squamous cell carcinoma of the cervix

Cervical cytology

→ 11.19 Normal cervical smear showing exfoliated cervical cells

Note the tiny nuclear remnants relative to the large volume of cytoplasm in each cell. (H & E stain; magnification x65.)

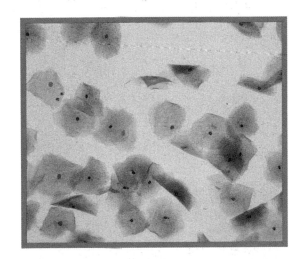

→ 11.20 Human papilloma virus

Numerous koilocytes can be seen. These cells show cytoplasmic vacuolation due to cytoplasmic necrosis. Occasionally, binucleate cells are also present.

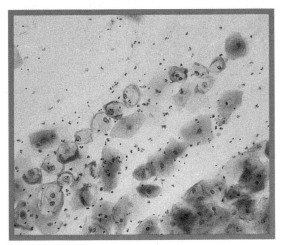

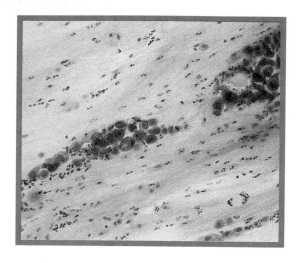

←11.21 Moderate dyskaryosis

Note that compared to the normal cells seen in **11.19** the abnormal cells are much smaller, but the nuclear/cytoplasmic ratio is approximately 50%. The nuclei vary in size and shape and chromatin distribution is irregular.

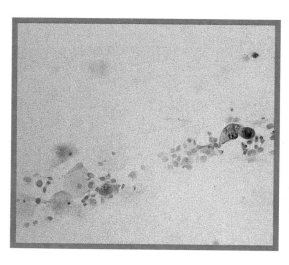

←11.22 Carcinoma cells

Note the very large nuclei with marked abnormality of the chromatin distribution and the very large nuclear/cytoplasmic ratio. (Magnification x65.)

12 | Lesions of the uterus and fallopian tubes

Developmental abnormalities

The uterus forms as the result of fusion of the two müllerian ducts. This process gives rise to the upper two-thirds of the vagina, the cervix, and the body of the uterus. A range of abnormalities may arise as the result of malfusion or non-development of the müllerian ducts. The most common abnormalities of the uterus include the following:
- The presence of a septum (subseptate uterus).
- Non-fusion of the two uterine horns to form a bicornuate uterus with a single cervix (**12.1–12.5**).

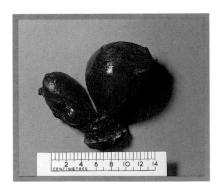

↑ 12.1 Bicornuate uterus

One horn is enlarged by a fibroid and there is a single cervix. Uterus bicornis unicollis.

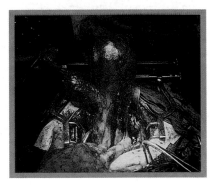

↑ 12.2 Bicornuate uterus

A further example of uterus bicornis unicollis.

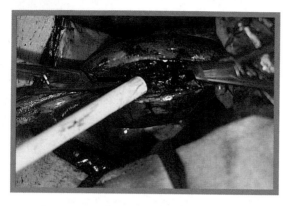

← 12.3 Bicornuate uterus: surgery

Metroplasty for unification of a bicornuate uterus. A transverse incision is made across the uterine fundus to expose the cavity of the uterus and the midline septum. Note that externally the uterine fundus appears normal.

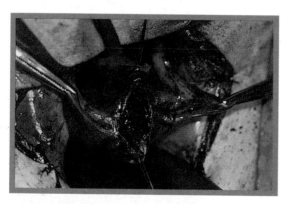

← 12.4 Bicornuate uterus: surgery

Once the septum is divided by diathermy, the uterine incision is closed anteroposteriorly.

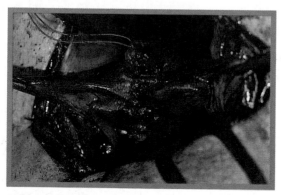

← 12.5 Bicornuate uterus: surgery

When closure of the uterus is complete, the cavity is enlarged anteroposteriorly. This ensures that the two cut surfaces of the septum do not adhere together.

Tumours

Tumours involving the body of the uterus arise either from the endometrium or the myometrium and may be benign or malignant (**12.6–12.19**).
- The most common benign tumours of the endometrium are endometrial polyps.
- The most common tumours of the myometrium are uterine myomas. Fibroids occur in approximately 20% of women over 30 years of age and in most women do not cause symptoms.

Approximately 67% of women with carcinoma of the endometrium present after the menopause. The peak age incidence is 65.4 years.

Malignant tumours of the myometrium are very rare and have a particularly poor prognosis. Tumours of the fallopian tubes are exceedingly rare and account for no more than 0.2% of all gynaecological malignancies.

→ 12.6 Uterine fibroid

Lower abdominal distension arising from a large uterine fibroid. The patient had a palpable mass in her lower abdomen, but was otherwise asymptomatic.

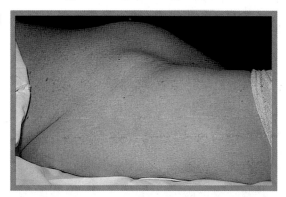

→ 12.7 Uterine fibroid

The grossly enlarged uterus is lifted out of the abdominal cavity at hysterectomy.

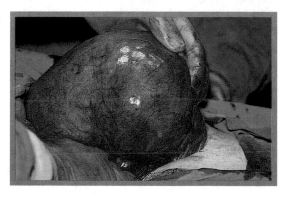

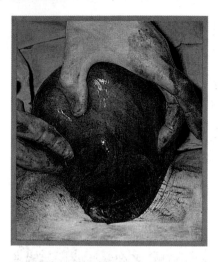

← 12.8 Uterine fibroid

The uterus is irregular because it contains multiple intramural fibroids.

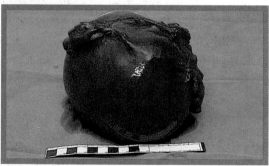

← 12.9 Uterine fibroid

The size of the uterus in this case can be seen in the final specimen.

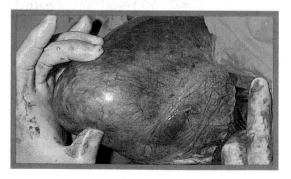

← 12.10 Multiple uterine fibroids

A further example of benign multiple uterine fibroids. This patient had severe menorrhagia.

→ 12.11 Multiple uterine fibroids

The ovaries in this case were also enlarged with multiple small cysts and the tubes were engorged and highly vascular.

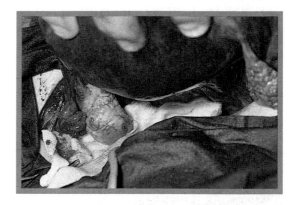

→ 12.12 Endometrial polyp

It is protruding through the cervical os.

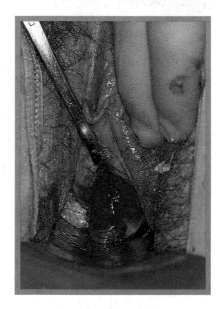

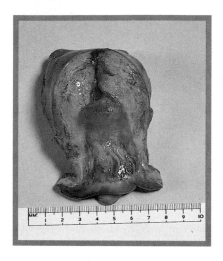

← 12.13 Submucous fibroid

This is contained within the cavity of the uterus and was causing menorrhagia and dysmenorrhoea.

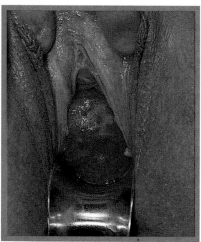

↑ 12.14 Fibroid polyp

This is protruding through the external cervical os, but arises from within the cavity of the uterus.

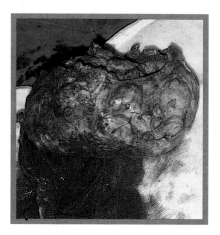

↑ 12.15 Large degenerating fibroid

This shows evidence of calcification.

→ 12.16 Large mixed müllerian duct tumour

These tumours are rare, but are generally highly malignant variants of uterine sarcomas.

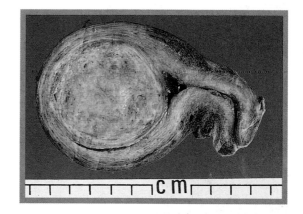

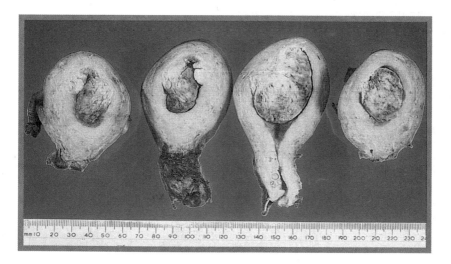

↑ 12.17 Large endometrial carcinoma

Multiple sections showing a large endometrial carcinoma invading the substance of the myometrium.

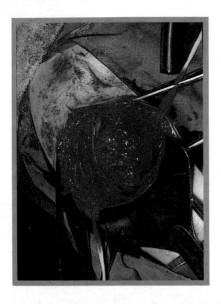

← 12.18 Hydatidiform mole

This photograph of a hysterectomy specimen was taken in 1965. It is now very rare to resort to hysterotomy for evacuation of molar tissue because most trophoblastic tumours are now removed by suction evacuation. The molar tissue can be seen filling the cavity of the uterus.

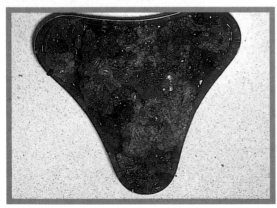

← 12.19 Hydatidiform mole

Dish containing the molar tissue after evacuation of the uterine cavity.

Endometriosis

Some aspects of endometriosis, particularly those deposits that arise outside the pelvic organs, are included in this chapter (**12.20–12.23**), while examples of ovarian endometriosis are included in Chapter 13.

→ 12.20 Endometriosis in a Caesarean section scar

The dark, tender mass at the left extremity of the wound becomes particularly painful and enlarged during menstruation.

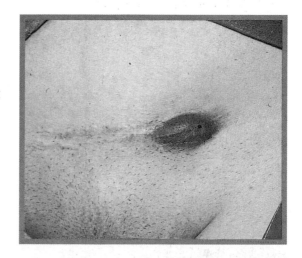

→ 12.21 Umbilical endometriosis

This patient bled from her umbilicus during menstruation. Superficial diathermy of the lesion in her umbilicus did not help and later it was necessary to excise the umbilicus. Intense scarring can be seen in the subumbilical tissue.

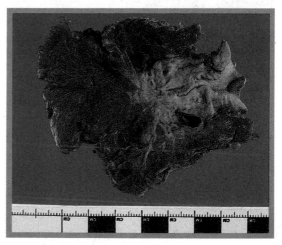

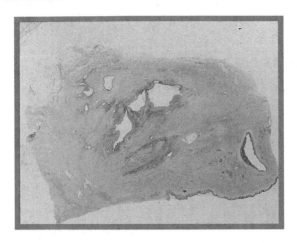

← 12.22 Umbilical endometriosis

A low power view of the H & E section shows active endometrial deposits within the scar tissue.

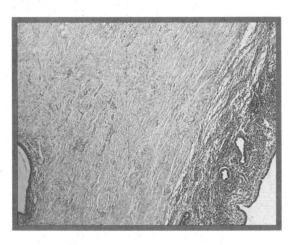

← 12.23 Umbilical endometriosis

Higher powered magnification shows the active epithelial lining of the cavity of the endometriotic deposits.

Lesions of the fallopian tube

The most common cause of tubal disease is bacterial infection. Acute salpingitis may result from sexually transmitted infection and the acute condition may progress to a state of chronic salpingitis and tubal obstruction (**12.24–12.28**). Carcinoma of the fallopian tube (**12.29**) is an exceedingly rare tumour which produces a "canary yellow" vaginal discharge and is often diagnosed late. Severe pelvic inflammatory disease is another cause of tubal lesions (**12.26–12.28**).

Tubal patency can be demonstrated radiologically by the injection of a radio-opaque dye through the cervix (**12.30**).

→ 12.24 Acute salpingitis

This shows the engorged swollen tubes associated with acute infection. The pelvis is relatively free of adhesions at this stage.

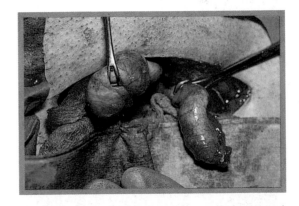

→ 12.25 Acute salpingitis

Beads of pus can be seen exuding from the fimbrial end of the tube.

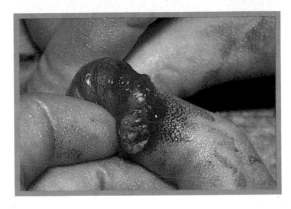

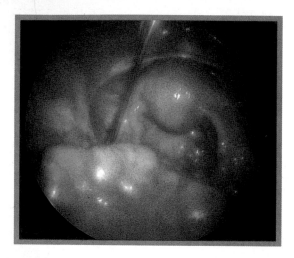

← 12.26 Chronic pelvic inflammatory disease

Laparoscopic view of the pelvis in chronic pelvic inflammatory disease. The pelvis is partly obscured by adherent bowel and omentum.

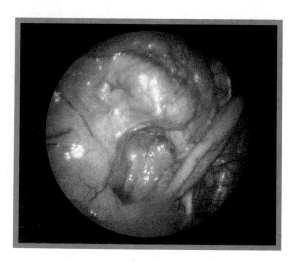

← 12.27 Chronic pelvic inflammatory disease

Omentum adherent over the right tube, which is swollen and occluded. The fimbrial ends of the tube have disappeared and this is now a hydrosalpinx.

→ 12.28 Chronic pelvic inflammatory disease

A sheet of fine adhesions cover the tubes and ovary, which is buried beneath the tube.

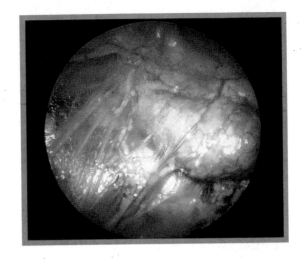

→ 12.29 Carcinoma of the fallopian tube

This is a rare tumour with a highly malignant potential. It generally presents late.

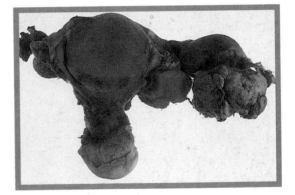

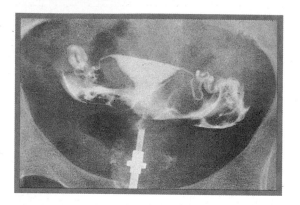

↑ 12.30 Evaluation of tubal function

This is performed either by insufflation with dye or radiologically, as shown here, by the injection of radio-opaque dye. The triangular outline of the uterine cavity can be seen and the spill of dye on both sides from the fimbrial ends of the tubes. The dye spreads over the adjacent bowel.

13 Lesions of
the ovary

The ovary is totipotential. Its structure varies on a cyclical basis and it produces the female sex hormones and the oocytes containing the genetic material of the mother. It is therefore not surprising that cystic and solid tumours of the ovary are common.

Ovarian lesions are commonly asymptomatic unless they undergo a complication such as torsion, rupture, haemorrhage, or necrosis. Signs of hormone-secreting tumours include virilisation or exaggerated female development, an abnormal menstrual cycle and precocious puberty.

Organic tumours of the ovary may be solid or cystic, benign or malignant. The ovary is also a common site of secondary tumours, particularly from primary sites in the breast and gastrointestinal tract.

Various examples of ovarian cysts, including those arising as a result of endometriosis, are demonstrated in **13.1–13.11.**

Follicular cyst

→ 13.1 Single follicular cyst

Cross section of a normal ovary showing a single follicular cyst near the surface of the ovary and close to the ovarian hilus.

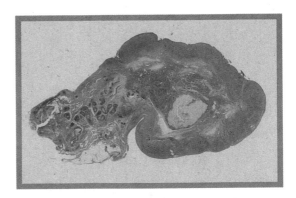

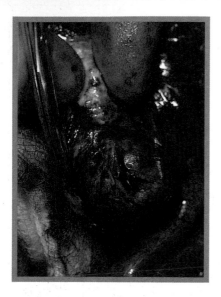

← 13.2 Small follicular cyst near mid-cycle

Surface appearance.

Endometriosis

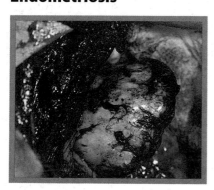

↑ 13.3 Endometriotic patches

Endometriotic patches on the surface of the ovary.

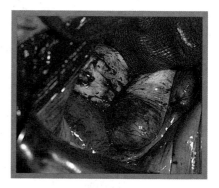

↑ 13.4 Bilateral ovarian enlargement

Both ovaries are affected by endometriosis and adherent behind the uterus.

→ 13.5 Ruptured endometrioma

Chocolate fluid from a ruptured endometrioma of the ovary.

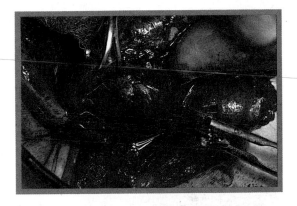

→ 13.6 Endometrioma

Intact endometrioma of the ovary removed with the uterus at hysterectomy.

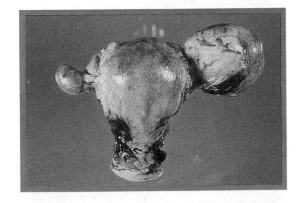

→ 13.7 Bilateral ovarian endometriomas

Removed at hysterectomy.

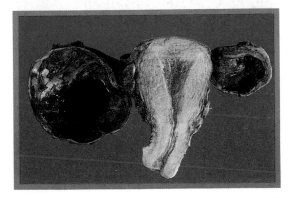

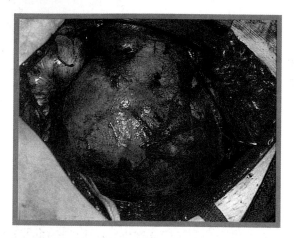

← 13.8
Endometriomatous 'plaque' on the uterine fundus

This is seen at the top side of this photograph with old altered blood on the adjoining surface.

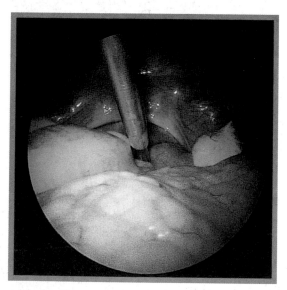

← 13.9
Endometriosis

Bowel and omentum adherent to the left ovary by endometriosis, identified at laparoscopy.

→ 13.10
Endometriosis

The same case as shown in **13.9**. An endo-metrioma can be seen on the left side in front of the ovary.

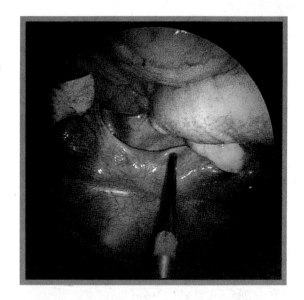

→ 13.11
Endometriosis

The probe demonstrates adhesions to the tube and ovary to the posterior leaf of the broad ligament.

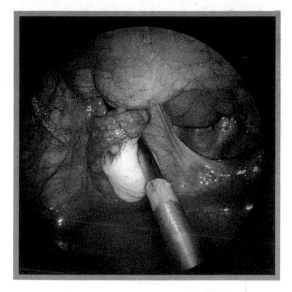

Benign cysts

Benign cysts of the ovary (**13.12–13.18**) are either functional or neoplastic.
- Functional cysts are rarely larger than 6 cm in diameter and are much more common than any other tumours of the ovaries. These cysts are follicular or lutein in origin and commonly occur in association with stimulation by gonadotrophins.
- Polycystic ovarian disease is associated with the presence of multiple small cysts in the ovary.
- Benign neoplastic tumours are epithelial in origin or arise from sex cord stroma or germ cell lines.
- Endometriotic cysts are common in the ovary.

All these benign lesions have malignant variants.

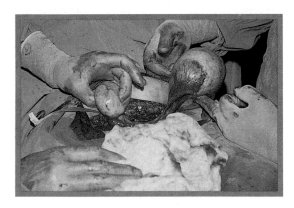

← 13.12 Bilateral dermoid cysts

Bilateral dermoid cysts demonstrated at laparotomy.

→ 13.13 Dermoid cyst

Contents of a benign cystic teratoma or dermoid cyst showing teeth and hair.

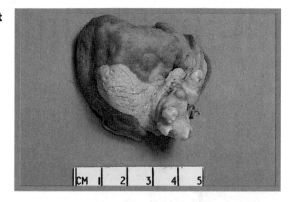

→ 13.14 Large benign ovarian serous cystadenoma

The tumour is shown at laparotomy.

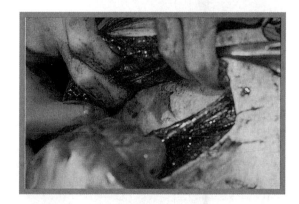

→ 13.15 Large benign ovarian serous cystadenoma

The tumour is delivered through the abdominal wound before removal.

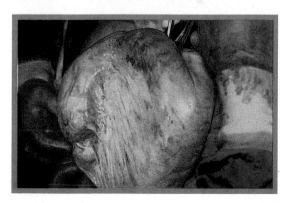

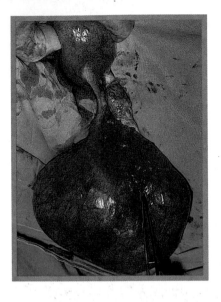

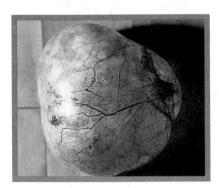

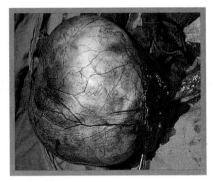

← 13.16 Large benign fimbrial cyst

The tube can be seen spread over the cyst.

↑ 13.17 Large benign fimbrial cyst

The fine vascular structure of the cyst wall is reinforced after reflection of the tube.

↑ 13.18 Large benign fimbrial cyst

Removal of the intact fimbrial cyst.

Malignant tumours of the ovary

The prognosis of malignant tumours of the ovary (**13.19–13.25**) is poor because spread is trans-coelomic and occurs as soon as the surface of the ovary is breached by the tumour. Carcinoma of the ovary accounts for 5% of all cancer deaths in women and the 5-year survival rate is only 25–30%. This is because 75% of such tumours present at an advanced stage.

Sex cord tumours are relatively rare (**13.26–13.31**) and are commonly hormone secreting. Androblastomas and Sertoli–Leydig cell tumours produce androgens and therefore exhibit signs of virilisation with increased facial hair, deepening of the voice and clitoral enlargement. On the other hand, granulosa cell tumours and thecomas produce oestrogen, and may cause precocious sexual development.

→ 13.19 Ovarian adenocarcinomas

Removal of bilateral malignant ovarian adenocarcinomas.

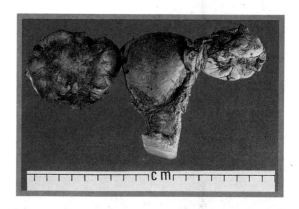

→ 13.20 Large endometrioid carcinoma of the ovary

The tumour is part cystic, part solid. The contralateral ovary is unaffected.

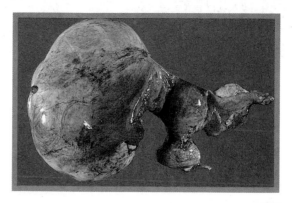

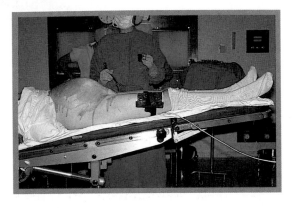

← 13.21 Large malignant ovarian tumour

Massive abdominal distension by a large malignant ovarian tumour.

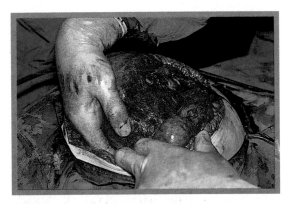

← 13.22 Advanced mucinous cystadeno-carcinoma of the ovary

Extensive omental tumour infiltrating from an advanced mucinous cystadenocarcinoma of the ovary.

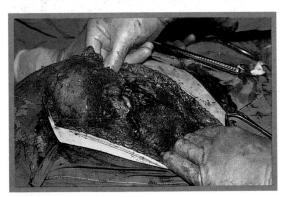

← 13.23 Advanced mucinous cystadeno-carcinoma of the ovary

Exposure of the tumour mass.

→ 13.24 Advanced mucinous cystadeno-carcinoma of the ovary

The final tumour specimen after excision.

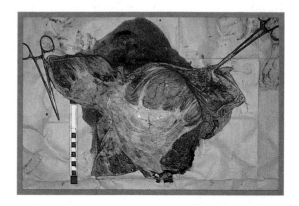

→ 13.25 Bilateral multicystic malignant ovarian tumours

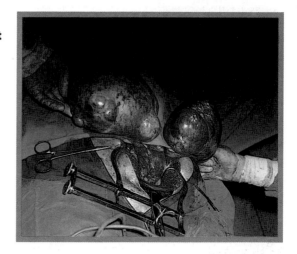

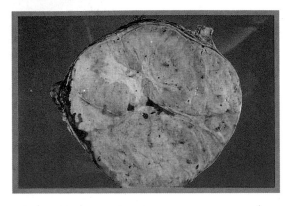

**← 13.26
Androblastoma or
Sertoli–Leydig cell
tumour**

Cross hemisection.
These tumours produce
testosterone and have
relatively low malignant
potential.

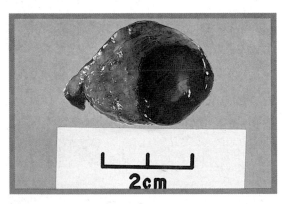

**← 13.27 A
Sertoli–Leydig cell
tumour**

About 50% of these
tumours produce
androgen and
virilisation.

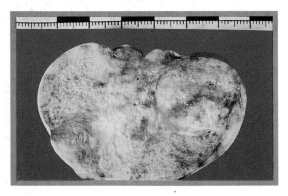

**← 13.28
Granulosa/theca cell
tumour**

This shows haemorrhagic
areas in the solid white
cut surface of the
tumour. These tumours
have low malignant
potential, with reported
5-year survival rates at
60–90%.

→ 13.29 A large thecoma or theca cell tumour

The cut surface is yellow, reflecting the presence of neutral lipid.

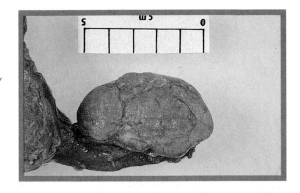

→ 13.30 Thecoma

Although thecomas are generally benign, if they secrete oestrogens they may cause, as in this case, an endometrial carcinoma. The thecoma can be clearly seen in the right ovary.

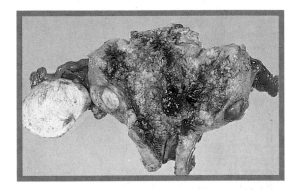

→ 13.31 Dysgerminoma of the ovary

These tumours have a solid, fleshy surface with a smooth lobulated exterior. The histological appearance is identical to that of a seminoma of the testis. The tumour is malignant, with a 5-year survival rate of 63% when it has extended beyond the ovary.

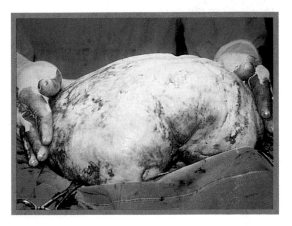

14 | Common gynaecological operations

It is important that those medical advisers who have a responsibility for counselling women with gynaecological disorders have some idea of what is involved in the commonly performed operations. This book is not a compilation of gynaecological procedures, but nevertheless, we feel that it is essential to include some pictures of the most commonly performed gynaecological operations. We therefore include descriptions of abdominal (**14.1–14.16**) and vaginal hysterectomy (**14.17–14.34**), dilatation and curretage (**14.35– 14.41**), diagnostic laparoscopy (**14.42–14.54**), open clip sterilisation (**14.55–14.57**), minimal invasive surgery (**14.58–14.66**) and laparascopic oophorectomy (**14.67–14.71**).

Abdominal hysterectomy

→ 14.1 Exposure of the right round ligament and broad ligament

The right side is anterior.

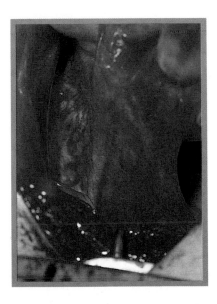

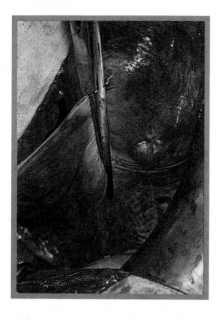

← 14.2 Placement of straight Kocher's forcep

Straight Kocher's forcep is placed across the fallopian tube to the left, the round ligament to the right, and part of the broad ligament.

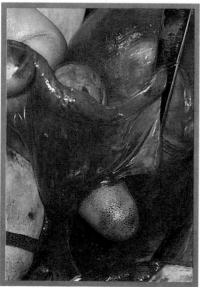

← 14.3 Division of the round ligament, isolation of the infundibulopelvic fold, division of the broad ligament

The round ligament is divided and the infundibulopelvic fold containing the ovarian vessels is isolated by pushing a finger through the broad ligament, which is then divided.

→ 14.4 The ovarian and round ligaments are transfixed and sutured

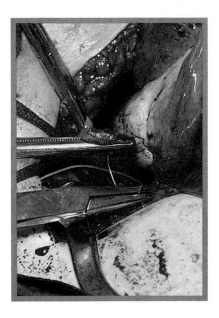

→ 14.5 Isolation of the lateral aspects of the uterine fundus

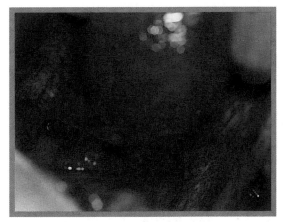

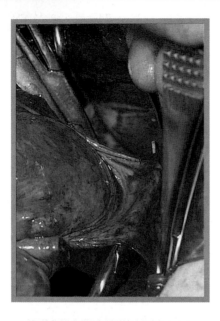

← 14.6 Dissection of the utero-vesical fold

The uterovesical fold of peritoneum is dissected free from the uterus and cervix.

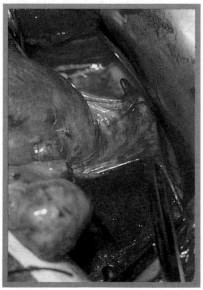

← 14.7 Division of the uterovesical fold

The uterovesical fold is divided with scissors on both sides of the uterus.

→ 14.8 Exposure of the uterine vessels

The uterine vessels are now exposed at the junction of the cervix and the body of the uterus.

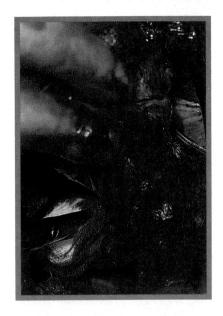

→ 14.9 Clamps are now applied across the uterine vessels

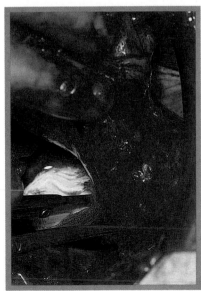

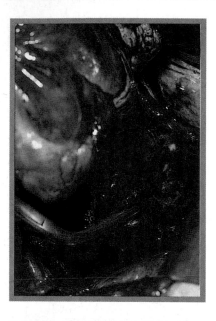

← 14.10 The clamps occlude all of the uterine vessels to the lateral margin of the uterus

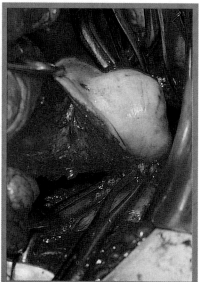

← 14.11 Division of the cardinal ligaments, opening of the vaginal vault

The cardinal ligaments are divided and the vaginal vault is opened to expose the cervix.

→ 14.12 After removal of the uterus

The uterus has now been removed and the pedicles and vaginal vault are sutured. Haemostasis is secured.

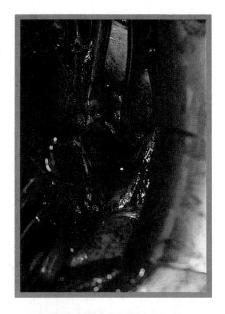

→ 14.13 After removal of the uterus

The rectum can be seen on the left and the sutures holding the round ligaments on the right.

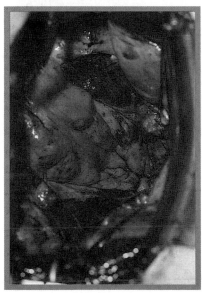

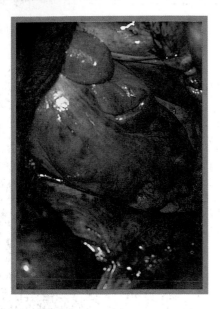

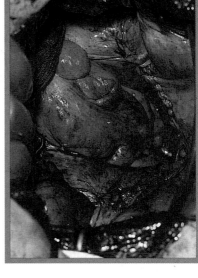

↑ 14.14 Closure of the pelvic peritoneum

↑ 14.15 The operation is now complete

The pelvic peritoneum is closed with a peritoneal suture.

← 14.16 The specimen

This consists of the uterus, tubes, and ovaries.

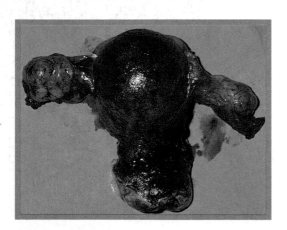

Vaginal hysterectomy

→ 14.17
Preparation of the patient

The patient is placed in the lithotomy position, cleaned, draped and catheterised.

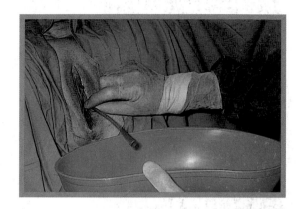

→ 14.18 The cervix is grasped with a vulsellum

The cervix is visible at the introitus and there is a visible cystocoele.

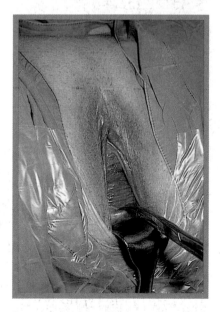

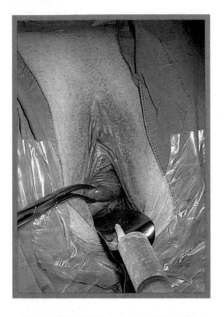

← 14.19 Infiltration of the para-cervical tissue

The paracervical tissue is infiltrated with saline with or without a vasoconstrictor.

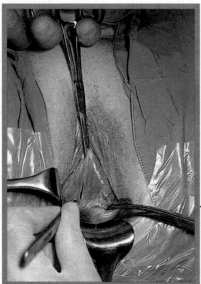

← 14.20 Freeing the bladder

A triangle of anterior vaginal wall is excised over the cystocoele and the bladder is dissected free.

→ 14.21 Demonstration of the enterocoele

The cervix is circumcised. The enterocoele is posterior to the cervix.

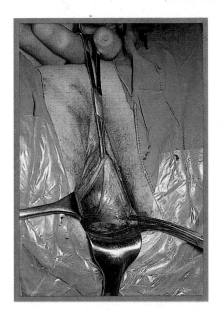

→ 14.22 Incision of the peritoneum

The peritoneum of the uterovesical fold is incised with scissors.

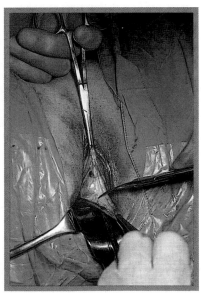

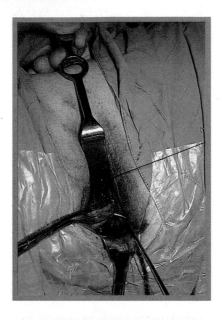

← 14.23 Insertion of a pedicle needle under the left cardinal ligament

The lateral cervical ligaments are exposed and a pedicle needle is inserted under the left cardinal ligament.

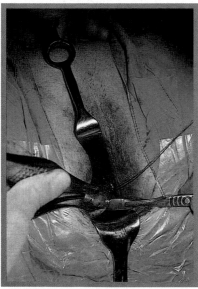

← 14.24 Separation of the cardinal ligament from the cervix

The cardinal ligament is cut until it is separated from the lateral aspect of the cervix.

→ 14.25 Exposure of the body of the uterus

The posterior peritoneum of the Pouch of Douglas is incised and the body of the uterus exposed.

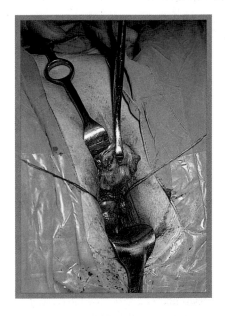

→ 14.26 The uterine vessels are clamped, cut, and transfixed

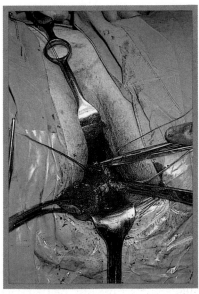

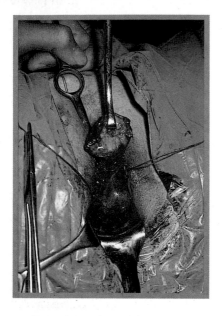

← 14.27 Descent of the uterine body

The uterine body, which contains several small fibroids, now descends.

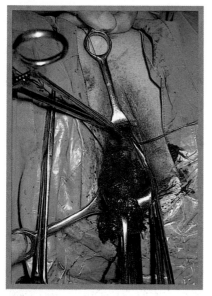

← 14.28 Cutting the pedicle

A clamp is applied across the round ligament, broad ligament, and fallopian tube, and the pedicle is cut.

→ 14.29 The uterine body and cervix are now delivered from the vagina

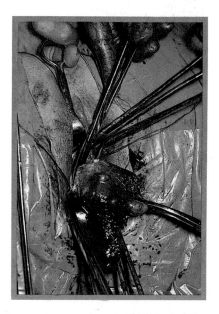

→ 14.30 Suturing the pedicles

The pedicles at the uterine horns are now sutured. The large bowel can be seen protruding through the peritoneal opening.

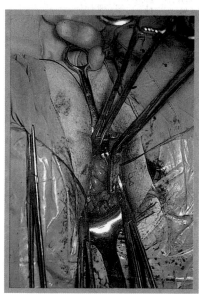

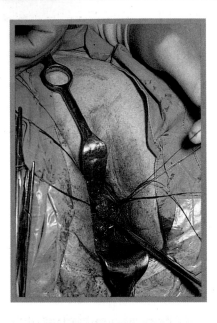

← 14.31 Closure of pelvic peritoneum

The pelvic peritoneum is now closed by cerclage, with exteriorisation of the pedicles.

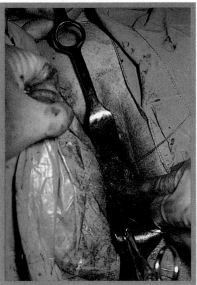

← 14.32 The pedicles are tied together at the vaginal vault

→ 14.33 The pedicles are tied to the vaginal vault

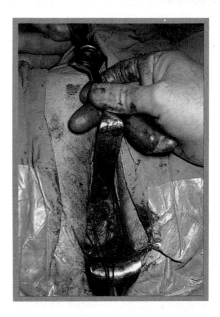

→ 14.34 Closure of the anterior vaginal wall

This is completed with interrupted sutures.

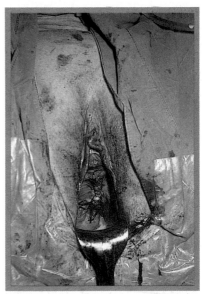

Dilatation of the cervix and endometrial curettage

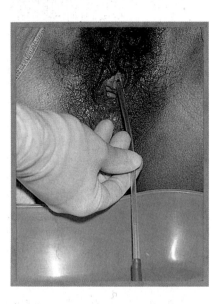

← 14.35 Preparation of the patient

The patient is placed in the lithotomy position, cleaned, draped, and catheterised.

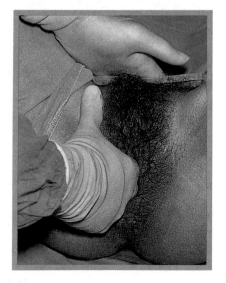

← 14.36 Preoperative observation

The position, size, shape, and mobility of the uterus are noted before the procedure is commenced.

→ 14.37 Exposure of the cervical os

A tenaculum is applied to the anterior lip of the cervix, a speculum is inserted, and the cervical os is clearly exposed.

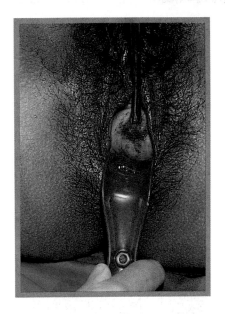

→ 14.38 Assessment of the uterus

The length and direction of the uterine cavity is measured and assessed with a sound.

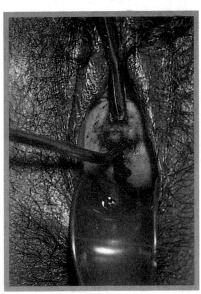

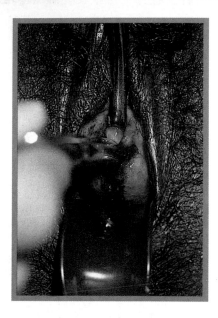

← 14.39 Dilatation of the cervix

The cervix is dilated by introducing progressively larger cervical dilators.

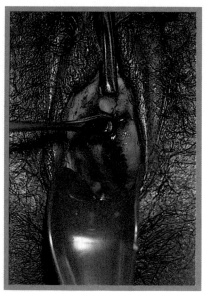

← 14.40 Removal of any polyps

Polyp forceps are introduced into the uterine cavity, opened, rotated, closed, and withdrawn to attempt to grasp and remove any polyps.

→ 14.41 Scrape of the uterine walls

A sharp uterine curette is inserted and the uterine walls are systematically scraped.

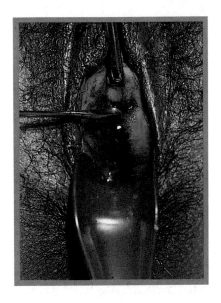

Laparascopy

→ 14.42 Preparation of the patient

The patient is draped and the bladder is catheterised.

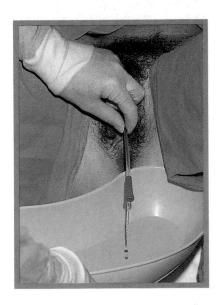

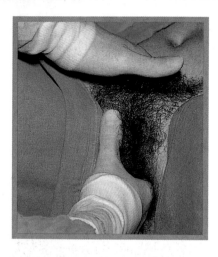

← 14.43 Vaginal examination

This is performed to determine the size and position of the uterus and whether there are any palpable adrenal masses.

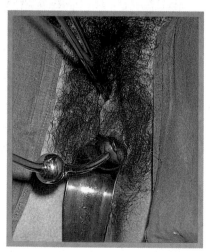

↑ 14.44 Insertion of a Spackman's cannula

The cervix is grasped with a tenaculum and a Spackman's cannula is inserted to manipulate the uterus.

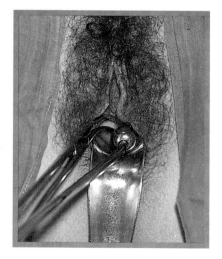

↑ 14.45 Insertion of a Spackman's cannula

The cannula is inserted to obtain a seal against the cervix.

→ 14.46 Making a small subumbilical incision

A small subumbilical incision is made before insertion of the Verres needle for insufflation of gas into the peritoneal cavity.

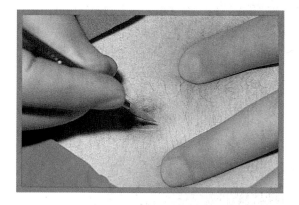

→ 14.47 Checking that the Verres needle is patent

The Verres needle is checked by gas insufflation to ensure that it is patent.

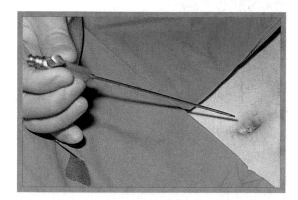

→ 14.48 Insertion of the Verres needle

The needle is inserted into the abdominal cavity and care is taken to ensure that it has not been inserted into the bowel or major blood vessels. The abdomen is then distended with 3–4 litres of carbon dioxide or nitrous oxide.

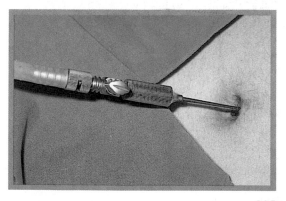

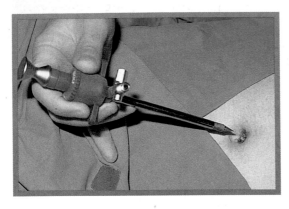

← 14.49 Insertion of the trocar

The trocar is inserted downwards towards the pelvic cavity.

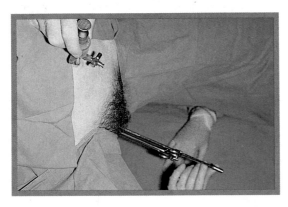

← 14.50 Visualisation of the pelvic organs

The uterus can now be manipulated to visualise the pelvic organs.

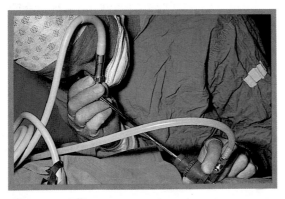

← 14.51 Insertion of a telescope

A telescope is inserted through the trocar and gas flow is sustained.

→ 14.52 Making a small suprapubic incision

A small suprapubic incision is made for introducing a probe to manipulate and display the pelvic organs.

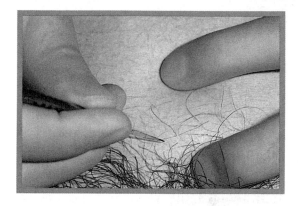

→ 14.53 Insertion of the suprapubic Steptoe probe

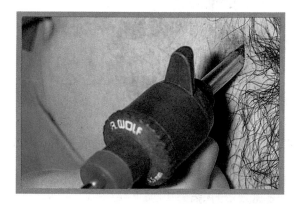

→ 14.54 Expelling the gas and suturing the wound

On completion of the procedure, the gas is expelled and the subumbilical wound is sutured.

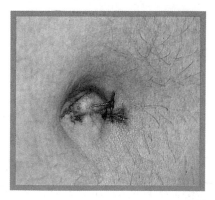

Open clip sterilisation

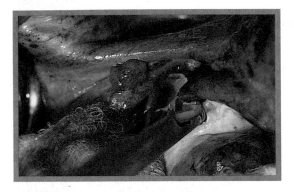

← **14.55 Application of a Filshie clip**

The right fallopian tube is grasped with the clip.

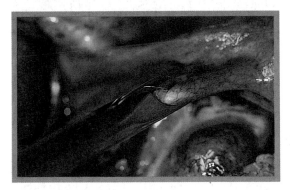

← **14.56 The clip is closed and the tube is crushed**

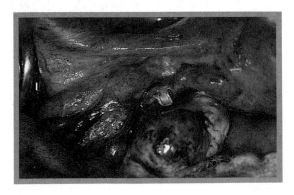

← **14.57 Filshie clip *in situ***

The Filshie clip is closed and locked across the fallopian tube.

Minimal invasive surgery

The advent of suitable instrumentation has led to the development of minimal invasive surgery, with many new techniques designed to gain access to the pelvic organs with small abdominal incisions. Two of the procedures—endometrial resection and ablation (**14.58–14.63**) and laparoscopic oophorectomy (**14.64–14.68**)—are described here as examples of these innovations.

→ 14.58 Endometrial resection and ablation

The patient is placed in the lithotomy position, cleansed, and draped, and the operating hysteroscope is introduced through the cervix.

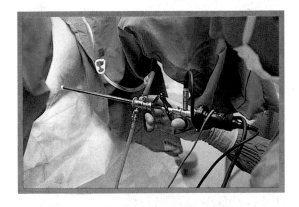

→ 14.59 Endometrial resection

After dilatation of the cervix, the resectoscope is inserted and the uterine cavity is distended with fluid. The endometrium is displayed on a television screen and the endometrium is resected.

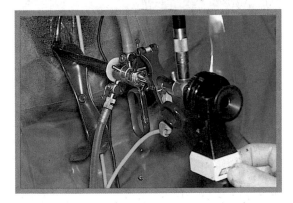

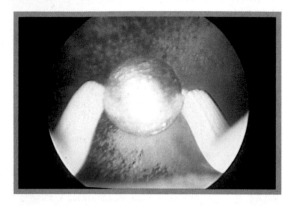

← 14.60 Endometrial resection and ablation

'Roller ball', used for diathermy, is placed inside the uterine cavity.

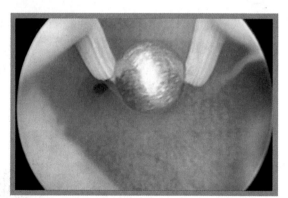

← 14.61 Endometrial resection and ablation

The ball is applied to the endometrium at the uterine fundus.

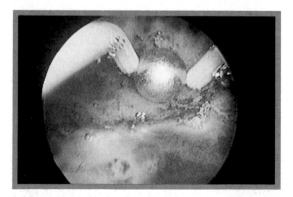

← 14.62 Endometrial resection and ablation

Diathermy of the endometrium in this fashion avoids preparation of the uterine fundus.

→ 14.63 Endometrial resection and ablation

Endometrial resection is performed elsewhere in the uterine cavity with loop excision of the endometrium and underlying myometrium.

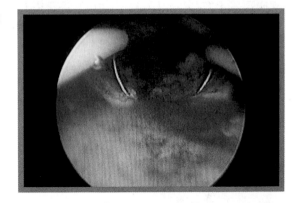

→ 14.64 Endometrial resection and ablation

Furrow created by loop excision.

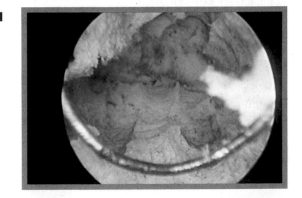

→ 14.65 Endometrial resection and ablation

End result of endometrial resection.

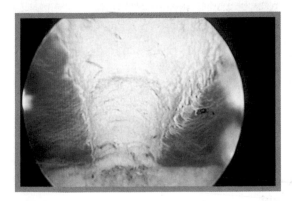

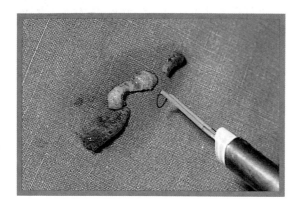

← 14.66 Endometrial resection

Strips of endometrium and underlying myometrium are resected and removed through the cervix.

Laparoscopic oophorectomy

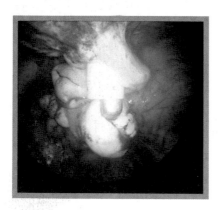

↑ 14.67 Laparoscopic oophorectomy

End of a large 10 mm grasper protruding through the cannula adjacent to the ovary.

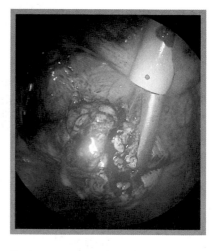

↑ 14.68 Laparoscopic oophorectomy

Grasper is applied to the ovarian pedicle.

**→ 14.69
Laparoscopic
oophorectomy**

Filshie clip is used as a
haemostat and applied
across the ovarian
pedicle.

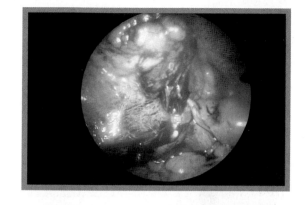

**→ 14.70
Laparoscopic
oophorectomy**

Preparation of the
pedicle for transsection
after application of the
Filshie clip.

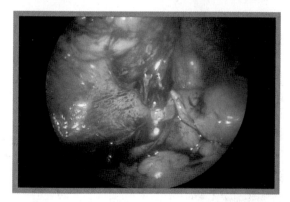

**→ 14.71
Laparoscopic
oophorectomy**

Pedicle divided with
removal of the ovary.

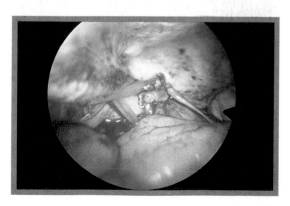

Index